BLACK BELT HUSBAND

A MARRIAGE BOOK FOR MEN

QUENTIN HAFNER, LMFT

Publishing Services provided by Paper Raven Books
Printed in the United States of America
First Printing, 2018

Paperback ISBN = 978-1-7324484-0-7
Hardback ISBN = 978-1-7324484-1-4

TABLE OF CONTENTS

This book is dedicated to all the men who work hard to show up everyday as great husbands. The world needs you today more than ever before. Never give up.

INTRODUCTION

Awakening to a 21st Century Paradigm of Being a Masculine Husband

THE CONFUSING ROLE OF THE MODERN HUSBAND

My friend, have you found yourself overwhelmed by the expectations placed upon you as a husband? Do you find these expectations foggy, and confusing? If so, you've landed in the right place.

Black Belt Husband provides a clear and actionable roadmap to help you gain clarity on how to be a successful husband in the twenty-first century. And not just any husband. Black Belt Husband is a journey about becoming a badass in marriage. Perhaps you're at a place in your own marriage where things don't seem to be going well. You may be fighting more or having less sex. Maybe you're just less satisfied than you've ever been. Or, you might even be one of many men who ended their marriage and want the tools and skills to be successful for another go around.

Whatever your reason for reading this book, I am convinced you won't be disappointed. There are a lot of confusing and conflicting messages about what it means to be a successful husband. How can you know what's right or wrong? Or good or bad? And how can you trust the source telling you the way you need to be?

We can be bombarded with messages that make us feel inadequate as husbands; like we're continually failing and not meeting others' expectations. Some of these messages come from our own wives while others may come from the therapists, counselors, and pastors we've turned to for help. To put salt on the wound, we get messages from a postmodern, radical feminist culture, that holds no punches in shaming men everywhere, working hard to convince us of our failures and inadequacies.

If you've felt confused or angry about some of this messaging, you're not alone. This book is for you. This book is not an attempt to change you or to limit your masculinity. In fact, it's quite the opposite. The contents of this book and the journey to Black Belt Husband are deeply masculine and you already have what it takes to get there. My job isn't to try and change you. My job, and the hope for this book, is twofold: to offer you a roadmap that helps you uncover your innermost masculine truth as a husband, and to fully access the love that you can offer your wife in your role as husband. You may have lost your way or you may have simply stumbled a little off the path. Either way, this book is a nudging to help you reclaim who you were meant to be in your role as husband.

MOVING FROM WHITE BELT HUSBAND TO BLACK BELT HUSBAND

In this book, I'm going to show you the traits necessary to be successful as a husband in the twenty-first century. All of these traits are timeless – they're the same qualities that our fathers and grandfathers bestowed on us. But they've been modernized to fit with the changing complexities of the twenty-first century. Becoming a Black Belt Husband is a developmental process. Meaning, we move through different stages represented by the belt ranking system, each of which lays the groundwork for success in the next stage. Much like the belt ranking system in martial arts, your ability to achieve the title of Black Belt Husband is determined by your successes with lower ranking belts.

The book is organized in sections that move us from white belt husbands to Black Belt Husbands. Our goal is to master the mindset and the associated skills with each belt, in order to move forward in the progression. As you progress toward Black Belt Husband, you'll learn how each of the attributes act as a foundation for being a successful modern husband. What's more, you'll be given the skills that need to be cultivated at each step of the way.

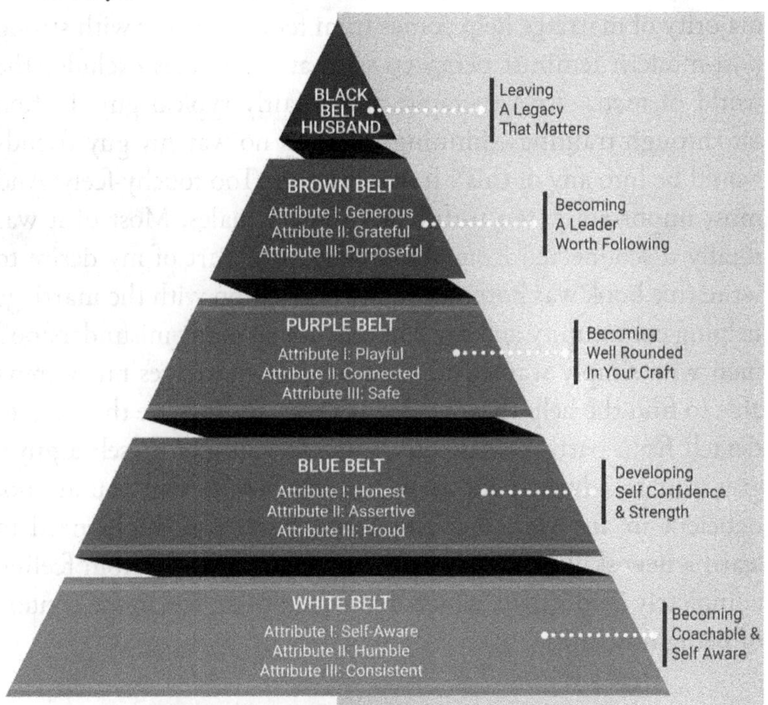

BLACK BELT HUSBAND HEIRARCHY

A MASCULINE VIEW OF MARRIAGE

Although I make no claims to be an expert in any martial art, I am a Brazilian jiu-jitsu practitioner, as well as a couples therapist with over 10,000 hours dedicated to counseling marriages and men just like you. The sport of Brazilian jiu-jitsu and the marriage journey share powerful parallels, and throughout the book I'll make references to them. I completely understand if martial arts isn't your thing. Don't let any of my comparisons and metaphors distract you from the real message of this book - the skills required to be a successful husband. You don't need to know anything about Brazilian jiu-jitsu to get a ton from this book.

When I became a couples therapist, I noticed early on that the profession was disproportionally female. In California, where I practice, the ratio of female to male therapists is four to one. The reason this is relevant is because the overwhelming majority of marriage help comes from females, many with strong post-modern feminist perspectives that sometimes excludes the world of men. As a therapist and a fairly typical guy, I often sat through trainings thinking, "There's no way my guy friends would be into any of this". It was too soft. Too touchy-feely. And most importantly, too unfriendly toward males. Most of it was totally disconnected from the average guy. Part of my desire to write this book was born out of my frustration with the marriage helping community and my empathy for so many misunderstood men who simply wanted to have happier marriages but weren't able to find the help they needed without feeling like they had to detach from part of their soul. I like to consider myself a guys-guy, and an advocate for men. I firmly believe that you are not deficient in any way, shape or form. Sure, you might need to learn a new skill here and there, but that's different from feeling completely inadequate, which many men often feel in the context of being husbands.

MY OWN BRUISES THROUGH THE JOURNEY

On a personal note, I've had to figure out marriage the hard way. I come from a family of multiple divorces where literally no one in my family knew how to do marriage well. This is not an indictment against my family, but simply a matter of fact. I was born into a family that taught me from a very early age how to fight horribly, how to be cold and distant, and how to run from your problems when things got difficult. Of course, there were some wonderful qualities about my family too, but when it came to core relationship skills, the most important things were missing. Solving relationship problems through compromising, negotiating, and while staying connected was something I never witnessed. My parents weren't bad people; they just didn't have the relationship skills to teach me something different. Their parents sadly did the same things with them and my parents just passed down what they were taught. Without a choice, I was born into the next generation of a lineage of broken families and marital disconnections.

As a kid, when my parents would fight, I would lie in bed feeling afraid and pray for them to divorce. I just wanted the yelling to stop. It was scary. As a child, I imagined my future as an adult and vowed that I would do things differently when I got married. I was certain that my story was going to be different.

During my twenties, I met and fell in love with someone. We dated for a few years and eventually married. From the beginning, our relationship was filled with instability, insecurity, and chaos. The dynamics of this relationship were very similar to those of my family. We fought horribly, we cheated on each other, and we created a marriage environment that was very unhealthy. We loved and cared about each other deeply, but we didn't have the skills to navigate the tumultuous waters of our relationship. Our care for each other wasn't enough. Eventually, amidst a mountain of emotional pain, we divorced.

In a post-divorce state of contemplation I asked myself: How was it possible that, despite my best efforts, I had just fallen into the same traps as my parents?

HOW COULD THIS HAPPEN?

Although as a child I swore to myself that I would have a different kind of marriage, I was troubled by the reality that I couldn't achieve it. I desperately wanted to understand what had just happened. One day, a friend mentioned therapy as a way to bring clarity to things. Of course the idea of talking about my feelings with a stranger sounded horrible, but I was humbled enough to entertain the idea. I didn't want my life to be a continual string of broken relationships, so I eventually found a therapist. It radically changed the trajectory of my life.

STARTING OVER AND BECOMING A THERAPIST

My experience in therapy was profound. I began taking a hard look at my past and seeing the generational patterns that had set me up for failure. I became aware of my fears in relationships and all of the defenses I used to keep people at a distance. I got more in touch with my painful childhood and the ways it negatively shaped my beliefs about marriage and relationships in general. In time, I came to a powerful conclusion about my relationships: I had zero chance at being successful in marriage unless I made some monumental changes.

After arriving at this realization, I was able to move away from blaming myself for the end of my previous marriage. I was also able to stop blaming other people. It wasn't my fault and it wasn't her fault. It wasn't my parents fault. There were no good guys or bad guys in this story, just two people who had literally no chance of making it work. What I came to see was that I was trying to run a marathon with two broken legs. In therapy, I learned that feelings of love alone are never enough to sustain a good relationship. I wrongly believed for years that feelings of love and affection carried good relationships. But feelings of love are never enough if you don't possess a baseline level of relationship skills. Skills I didn't have. And skills that I see many men in my therapy practice not having. Gradually over time, I discovered this missing set of skills that I hadn't previously been taught. It's these skills, a new mindset, and a totally different understanding of marriage that I want to share with you in this book.

HELPING MEN LEARN A NEW WAY IN RELATIONSHIPS

My personal experience in therapy and my wanting to make my own relationships successful catapulted me into graduate school to study marriage and family therapy. Before I applied to graduate school, I had a great career and I never imagined I would be a therapist. I wasn't really the type of guy who would become a therapist. Truly. But there was something so compelling about wanting to share the information I learned and the experience I had with other men just like me. It drove me to leave my career and head down the path of becoming a couples therapist.

I felt strongly that if I could just spare one other guy from having to live through the horrendous pain of a broken marriage, it would all be worth it. That was the beginning of my journey. My co-workers thought I had lost my mind when I told them I was becoming a therapist.

I finished graduate school, got licensed as a therapist, and began building a practice to help married guys in relationships. I read everything I could on the subject. I went to workshops, did extensive post-graduate trainings, continued in my own therapy, and consulted with the best couples experts I could find to deepen my understanding of relationships.

As I began working with more men, I saw that even those who grew up in more stable families often lacked the necessary understanding and relationship skills needed to make marriages work in the twenty first century. Even though they didn't come from chaotic families like I did, they weren't immune to failed marriages. Many of these men came from good families, but their marriages were falling apart too. They were always shocked when this happened. I learned that none of us are immune, and regardless of our background and upbringing, marriage is a more complex relationship than it was in prior generations. This book sheds light on how we can adapt to these changing complexities. We can learn to take what was good from our family of origin and leave behind what won't work anymore.

With this new paradigm of what it takes to make marriages work and a new relationship skillset to draw upon, I am now remarried to the most spectacular woman. Of course, our relationship has its own share of challenges, but a critical difference is that challenges are easily overcome and moved through. No longer are there hills to die on. We may disagree with each other, but we remain deeply connected. We may mistakenly hurt each other, but know how to repair these moments. We're honest with one another and we help each other get the most out of life. We genuinely want the best for one another.

The relationship success I've experienced has come from lots of hard work and lots of self-reflection. As you enter into this journey toward becoming Black Belt Husbands, I want you to know that I come to the table with my own failures and setbacks. I want to share them with you, as a way to remind you that it's not about good relationship genes. It's a learning-process that's available to anyone. I had to go about it the hard way, but you can do it differently. You can adopt the right frame of mind and learn the necessary skills that took me decades to figure out both personally and professionally. That's what this book is about. It's the roadmap that I never had and most guys never have. I simply want to share with you what I've learned.

WHAT WE'LL LEARN ALONG THE WAY

This book can help you unlock a great marriage. It outlines the how and why behind being an irresistible husband while recognizing you can, and need to, hold on to your inherent masculinity. If you really digest this book and implement the strategies provided, you are divorce-proofing your marriage. And even beyond not getting a divorce, the contents in this book can help you be truly happy in your marriage and with yourself as an individual.

This book is not about fixing your wife and making her better. This is about looking at you, the husband. Still, I'm confident that applying the books contents will bring responses from her that you didn't think were possible anymore. With that said, it's not about her problems or the things she needs to do differently. It's about looking at ourselves and recognizing that the only thing we can change is us. When we have this realization, we are finally free. Unshackled from the burden of worrying about and focusing on someone else. This book is a journey into yourself and becoming the man you were created to be. It's about harnessing your inborn masculine spirit, which produces a well-balanced, healthy male with lots of self-confidence, power, strength, and relationally intelligent qualities. When you become this type of person - a Black Belt Husband - marriage flows smoothly and setbacks are easily course-corrected. As we go through the twelve attributes of the belt ranking hierarchy toward Black Belt Husband, each chapter will be organized in the following way:

i. What does this particular attribute look like for a Black Belt Husband
ii. Why is this particular attribute essential for success
iii. Typical problems that arise for men who are missing this attribute
iv. What does this attribute have to do with healthy masculinity

v. Questions you can ask yourself to assess your progress with this attribute
vi. Practical solutions to improve this attribute
vii. The tangible benefits to your relationship when you gain more of this attribute
viii. The practical skills needed to move on toward the next rank

Each chapter and attribute will leave you with the two essentials ingredients for personal developmental gains: knowledge and practical action steps. With these two elements, you'll be able to move through the book with new understandings and steps that can be taken toward improvement. You will have what you need to know and do in order to move to higher ranks. No more feeling lost or overwhelmed by a myriad of conflicting societal messages. You'll have what you need at all times.

WHAT'S WAITING FOR YOU ON THE OTHER SIDE

Similar to Brazilian jiu-jitsu black belts, Black Belt Husbands are rare. You can't buy a black belt as a husband any more than you can buy one in Brazilian jiu-jitsu. You can only earn one through consistent dedication, practice, and training.

Black Belt Husbands are not born, they are made through trials, successes, and a continual refinement process. If you work toward becoming a Black Belt Husband, you have so much to gain. For starters, you will fight less, have more sex, and feel much more peaceful in your relationship. You will have more fun, and your wife will be friendly with you. That is the promise of this book. If you value your marriage and are looking to be happier moving forward, this book is for you.

Before we get into the contents of the book, I want you to take a second to fill out a quick relationship questionnaire. It's a simple, twenty-question assessment that measures your current standing on the Black Belt Husband journey. It shouldn't take more than sixty seconds to complete. When you're done with the book and after you've implemented the action steps, I want you to take the survey again to see your improvement and your current ranking. My promise to you is that your relationship satisfaction will have greatly improved. It's a fun and direct way to see your growth.

Please visit: www.BlackBeltHusband.com

IT'S GO TIME

If you're in a marriage that feels a little rocky, please don't delay in reading and implementing the material in this book.

Unfortunately, time is not our friend in these scenarios.

Sadly, I've worked with too many men who were shocked and devastated when they were presented with divorce. If your marriage hasn't been strong in some time, it's time to take action. You owe it to yourself to act in advance. Statistically, 70 percent of all divorces are initiated by women. And I can attest that many, many men had no idea it was coming. But we don't have to be part of those statistics. We have free will and a desire for something greater. Take action and begin the journey toward Black Belt Husband. There is so much to gain by participating in this experience. Please don't regret waiting. As you begin the journey in this book, I strongly encourage you to read it slowly, bit by bit, and journal along the way. Don't just devour the contents mindlessly. Grab a journal, a pen, and take notes along the way. You will get much more out of it this way. My friend, let's get started with Section One – the White Belt Journey.

SECTION ONE

The White Belt Journey; Being Coachable and Open-Minded

Make no mistake, you earn a white belt. The belt is a physical representation of a commitment to the beginner's mind. It is a vulnerability and a willingness to learn that shines through.

—Chris Matakas, *The Tao of Jiu Jitsu*

GETTING READY FOR THE WHITE BELT JOURNEY

The white belt journey is an exciting one. It's filled with renewed hope about the future and a lot of self-discovery. Similar to the white belt journey in the martial arts, the white belt journey toward Black Belt Husband is not the most sexy or alluring stage of the journey. It's humbling, and it's grounding. It symbolizes you are a beginner. But it's essential that you master the fundamentals before you can move to more complex tasks that await you in higher ranks.

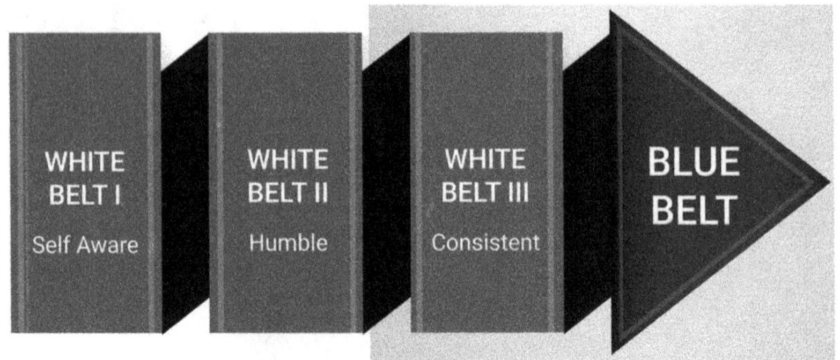

CHAPTER 1

White Belt I: Self-Aware; Boldly Knowing Ourselves

DIGGING DEEP TO KNOW OURSELVES

What if I asked you a simple question: Can you tell me three things you do that get in the way of having a better marriage? I know you could rattle off a long list of what she does, but can you do the same for yourself? It might seem like a simple question, but it can be difficult to answer unless you've really spent some time thinking about it. This is an example of self-awareness; the beginning of the road toward Black Belt Husband.

Self-awareness is the degree to which we know ourselves: the good, the bad, and the ugly. It's an understanding of our strengths and weaknesses. Sometimes referred to as insight, self-awareness consists of knowing our patterns of interaction in relationships, the origin of those patterns, and our life experiences that have influenced them. The importance of having a baseline level of self-awareness can't be overstated. Without it, we'll continually stumble over our own feet in marriage. We have to get to know ourselves - our thoughts, our emotions, our perceptions, and our behaviors.

Gaining a greater degree of self-awareness is about having a more clear picture of *why* we do what we do. When we gain more self-awareness, it's like we discover a new roadmap that helps us make sense of our path, instead of mindlessly driving around lost in the middle of the night. The black belt in Brazilian jiu-jitsu is incredibly self-aware; so too are Black Belt Husbands. Black Belt Husbands know themselves - the attributes that make them successful and the things that get in their way. Without this kind of self-knowledge, we will not have a way to navigate difficult relationship scenarios. The more we grow in self-awareness, the more we can make sense of these difficult scenarios in a way that doesn't leave us hopelessly stuck.

WITHOUT SELF-AWARENESS, WE CAN'T MOVE FORWARD

The foundation for any great relationship is built upon two people developing an adequate amount of self-awareness throughout the course of their relationship. The great philosophers and wisdom writers were saying it thousands of years ago; "Know thyself!" It holds true for us today as much as it did then. There is a reason the smartest humans throughout history kept talking about it; its importance for the Black Belt Husband journey can't be understated. Gaining a foundational level of self-awareness is white belt work because so much of the work in higher ranking belts depends upon it. Still, the work of self-awareness doesn't stop with the white belt; it is a lifetime undertaking.

A good example to illustrate the value of self-awareness is the guy who comes home from work after his boss berates him for making an error on the job. He walks through the front door of his home pissed off and kicks the dog. When his wife asks him, "Why did you kick the dog?" the man replies, "That stupid dog is always in the way!" We understand in this cliché story that the man's anger wasn't really about the dog, but about what happened at his work. He didn't have the self-awareness to realize it. In this story, the man kicks the dog, but in many other stories, the man might come home and snap at his wife. He might yell at his kids or retreat into his own personal cocoon of isolation and withdrawal. Not exactly sure why he's doing any of this. Our goal is to become increasingly aware of the thoughts and emotions that drive our behaviors.

WHEN LIMITED INSIGHT BECOMES OUR ACHILLES HEEL

Throughout my work with men in my counseling practice, I've come to appreciate and respect that men are very much action oriented. We are hard-wired to be "doer's". We are problem-solvers and fixers. Society at large enjoys the comforts that have been built upon the hard work and action-oriented achievements of great men. So, if you're anything like me, you probably have a bias toward action and doing versus the contemplative nature of "being" that is required to gain greater levels of self-awareness.

I get it.

I really do.

I'm a doer myself and generally loathe sitting still for too long without taking action. I usually feel like I have a million things to do and a million places to be. But this can also be my Achilles heel. I often trip over myself because I have a hard time slowing down. Developing greater insight requires that we slow down a bit. We must not be in too much of rush. We have to be still for a little while and think things through. We live in a hyper-fast world that is not conducive to more self-reflection. Particularly with the advent of smart phones, it's critical that we're intentional about letting our minds think through and process things. I understand this attitude flies in the face of our action-oriented preferences.

I've worked with a few different black belts getting private lessons in BJJ. I was always struck by the fact that all of them encouraged me to take notes and journal after our private lessons. They wanted me to take time to write down what I had learned, and spend time in self-reflection thinking about it. They said that my success and growth was dependent upon that. They asked me to visualize the techniques and concepts outside of class. These coaches knew that self-reflection was as important as the actual physical aspect of the sport if I was to make real progress.

In BJJ improvement is a two-part process: the doing (mat time) and the thinking (gaining more insight). Becoming a Black Belt Husband works exactly the same way. It's a combination of self-understanding and taking the right steps in action. When we don't have a baseline level of self-awareness, we run the risk of getting stuck in our relationships by failing to take responsibility for ourselves. It's easy to get stuck believing our partner is the problem and disavow our own contribution. This tendency to look outward instead of inward usually happens to men who have limited insight. The good news is that self-awareness is an attribute that can be learned and grown over time.

IT'S NOT HER, IT'S ME

I don't know about you, but have you ever noticed how annoying it feels to be around someone who continually blames others for all of their struggles in their life? Everything wrong about their world is because of someone else, their bad luck, or the cosmos is simply against them. You've met people like this, right? These types of people are great examples of those who don't have much self-awareness. They can't see how their own actions, behaviors, and thoughts contribute to their demise. The problem is always outside of them. But in reality, their problems are not about everyone else. Their problems are often due to their own actions, decisions, and behaviors.

Well, marriage problems aren't any different. Whenever problems arise in marriage, the knee-jerk reaction for most of us is to blame our partner. We see her as the problem, instead of seeing how we contribute to what's happening. Now I'm not saying that your wife is without fault; of course she totally blows it too. But that's too easy. It's much harder to look at ourselves. What we're trying to think about here is how well we can identify and acknowledge *our* contribution. When we achieve a baseline level of self-awareness, we're able to step outside of ourselves and generally see that blaming others for our challenges will get us nowhere. Literally. It will just keep you stuck. Insight helps us see how we are a part of the problem and it allows us an opportunity to take responsibility for our part, without the need to blame others.

Being successful in this section is learning how to fight with yourself.

Learning how to wrestle with your own demons.

Learning to look inward instead of outward.

This is something that I continue to work on personally and something that I was really bad at for most of my adult life. I used to feel absolutely certain that my reactions were because *of* something someone else did. I know now that only I am responsible for my reactions. Although I don't have it perfected, I realize I have to be open to take responsibility for my emotions and my behaviors without assuming that it *was because of* something my wife did. Blaming others for your actions is not the way of the mature masculine man.

When we become more insightful, we're receptive to criticism because we can view it as a tool that helps us shape our lives for the better. We're a lot less defensive around criticism because we've already established a baseline level of knowing ourselves –our strengths and our weaknesses. People that are more self-aware don't experience criticism as a personal affront to their character because the criticism is either true or it's not true.

We already know what is true because we know ourselves. So, if someone says, "Hey, I think you need to work on that thing....", we can say, "Yeah, you're right ... that thing is a sticking point for me" if it rings true. If we don't know ourselves enough and don't have enough insight, there's a good chance that we're going to respond defensively because the criticism is going to feel like an assault on our character. Mature masculinity can tolerate criticism without feeling compelled to fight back. Self-awareness helps us get to this place.

But when we know ourselves, we can recognize a criticism for just what it is: another person's perspective on us that's either accurate, or inaccurate. When we don't know ourselves, all criticism feels inaccurate, and we respond defensively from this place. Becoming a Black Belt Husband means having enough insight to be able to discern when someone's criticism of you is wrong and knowing when their criticism is right.

HOW WOULD YOU RATE YOUR LEVEL OF SELF-AWARENESS?

Let's take a look at some questions you can use to assess your level of self-awareness. The list of questions we could ask is literally infinite, so for now, I'm keeping it focused on establishing a baseline level of insight. As we move into later chapters and up the ranks, our insight will become stronger. As we get into these questions, it's very important that you understand we are not judging ourselves or condemning our answers. This is simply an exercise in self-awareness, not any kind of indictment of our character.

QUESTIONS TO ASSESS YOUR LEVEL OF SELF-AWARENESS

- What were your father's top three positive attributes as a husband when you were young?
- What were your father's top three deficits as a husband when you were young?

- When you feel stressed out, what is your healthy coping mechanism?
- When you feel stressed out, what is your unhealthy coping mechanism?
- What stresses are you currently dealing with that are impairing your marriage?
- In the face of fear, overwhelm, or stress, do you fight or do you flee?
- And what does fight or flee look like for you practically?
- What is your greatest fear about marriage and being a husband?
- What do you think is your greatest asset as a husband?
- What is your greatest deficit as a husband?
- When it comes to conflict, are you a "rager" or do you shut down?
- What does your wife not know about you that you wish she did?
- What life events have caused you to not trust others?

BLACK BELT HUSBAND TRAINING: DEVELOPING MORE SELF-AWARENESS

You may have answers to these questions and feel as though you've already developed some clarity around them. Awesome. Others may read this bulleted list and think, "Oh wow, is this stuff really that important? This sounds like a bunch of psychobabble bullshit". Reader, if this is you, please hang with me and allow me to show you why this stuff really matters. By no means is self-awareness by itself going to give us the marriage of our dreams, but it's one of the critical ingredients to get us there. When it comes to developing more insight, there are a few tried and true ways that can get us where we need to be fairly fast.

Method #1: Journaling

Spending time alone journaling through the above questions can be massively helpful in developing more self-awareness. There's something powerful about paper and pen and writing down our thoughts and our perceptions in an undistracted setting. If you want to achieve Black Belt Husband, you're going to have to get comfortable with spending some time in solitude in order to think through what's happening. There's no other way to accomplish greater levels of self-awareness.

Method #2: Letting People Speak Truth to You

If you're brave enough, you can ask someone that's close to you how they would answer some of these questions - as they see you. Sometimes, we have blind spots and it's hard to see ourselves accurately. Asking people how they see us, can be very helpful in jump-starting the process. You can even take the list of questions above and ask five friends how they would answer for you. For example, if I ask four close friends how they see me as a husband, and I get some common-denominator answers, well then, maybe there's a good chance some it is true. Ask those closest to you how they see you. Ask those who are closest to you for input on your greatest strengths and weaknesses.

Method #3: Finding a Good Counselor

Finding a good counselor can be the greatest gift you ever give yourself. There's something powerful about having someone in your life that can help you develop a lens of objectivity. Friends and family are great, but they are often biased in their perceptions of us. Personal development work through therapy affords us the opportunity to take a look at some of the things we struggle with in a non-judgmental, but honest environment. Sometimes that type of relationship can be hard to find in our lives outside of therapy.

THE BENEFITS OF BECOMING MORE SELF-AWARE

Having a baseline level of self-awareness is foundational white belt stuff because so much of the higher-ranking belts are dependent upon our ability to honestly reflect about ourselves. We have to know where we stand on certain spectrums or continuums of personality and behavior in order to make change in the right direction. Insight helps us to know where we're at on the map. Growing in insight is a lifelong process, just like learning jiu-jitsu. We never really master it, we just become better over time with greater levels of confidence. When we grow in self-awareness, our marriages benefit because:

- We're less defensive in our arguments, which typically ends arguments quicker.
- We can push back against inaccurate perceptions without getting offended or needing to fight back.
- We become more confident around other people, which typically makes us more captivating.
- We're less boring and more fascinating to others. Our increased self-awareness can lead to more frequent and better sex because our partners will develop a great attraction to us.
- We become more active participants in our marriages because we can share about ourselves. We will never hear, "You never say anything about yourself".

WHITE BELT SKILLS TEST

PRACTICAL SKILL NEEDED TO MOVE FORWARD

Approaching relationships with a mindset that none of us are perfect and all of us can improve, what is the ONE BIG THING that you feel you need to change about yourself in order to be more effective in your role as husband? Can you clearly identify that? At this point in the journey, we simply want to have clarity around the most apparent and predictable stumbling block that might get in the way of a great marriage.

- Is it that you get angered too easily?
- Maybe you're not present enough?
- Maybe you're too nice and too much of pushover?
- Maybe she would say that you work too much?
- Maybe you've stopped prioritizing yourself?
- Maybe you drink too much?
- Maybe you avoid her instead of engaging with her?

Required Skill: Identifying Your ONE THING

At this point, I simply want you to think through the questions above and identify what that one thing is. Write it down.

Once you arrive at that thing, I want you to identify three little things you can commit to right now to start changing this. Write those down too.

This is where we get to take action. I simply want you to start doing something right now to begin changing the tide. No more stagnation. If you commit to working on this, combining more self-awareness with positive action, I can promise you that when combined with challenges set forth in later chapters, your marriage will go through an incredible overhaul. Your willingness to take action with the small changes is what's going to get you to Black Belt Husband.

CHAPTER 2

White Belt II: Humble; Being Brave Enough to Not Know

HAVING ENOUGH CONFIDENCE TO BE OK NOT HAVING IT ALL TOGETHER

Being successful in marriage without lots of humility is simply impossible. Spend a little time talking to any couple that has been happily married for many years, and one of the first things you'll notice is the humility. When we have too much ego, pride, and insecurity to keep us from admitting our frailties, we are destined for relationship demise.

Brazilian jiu-jitsu is very similar. This sport has a miraculous way of taking the most arrogant person and giving them a dose of humility that is destined to change them. It's the most humbling sport I've ever experienced, rivaled only by the marriage journey. Marriage is very humbling if we allow it to be. But we often resist humility because we struggle to see its benefits. Sometimes, we can be too stubborn to learn a new way or to absorb the life lessons that marriage wants to teach us. Being humble as a marriage partner is foundational to Black Belt Husband because we have to remain open to learning and seeing things from a different perspective. We have to approach marriage with the recognition that we don't know what we don't know. We have to see the paradox, and embrace the truth that humility is a sign of true strength. Conversely, the lack of humility is the ultimate reflection of insecurity.

I remember this one guy who came to his first introduction class at my jiu-jitsu academy. He was huge guy, about 6'4" and shredded with muscle. He was tattooed from head to toe and looked really intimidating. He was the stereotypical tough guy. After a few minutes sparring with a much smaller, but skilled opponent for a couple of rounds, this guy came face-to-face with the sobering reality that his size and strength didn't mean as much as he thought it meant. On his first day, he was submitted time after time, barely able to come up for air. Over the course of the next several months, I watched this guy's attendance in class wane. After about twelve weeks, he eventually quit and never returned. Sadly, this guy's ego, pride, and identification with being a tough guy were challenged. And instead of embracing the challenge humbly and welcoming an incredible opportunity to learn something new, he walked away.

Marriage is very similar. It will test us and challenge our pride. Marriage will submit us. If we don't approach marriage with a willingness to learning new ways of engaging, the journey will eventually break us.

WITHOUT HUMILITY, WE STAND NO CHANCE

After my divorce with my first wife, it became painfully clear that I had no idea what I was doing in marriage. Unfortunately, I needed to experience a painful setback with my divorce before

I could submit to marriage with a sense of humility. I resisted at first, but I eventually accepted that I honestly had no idea how to be a successful husband. I went through a period where I blamed my ex-wife, but eventually I had to come face-to-face with my own shortcomings. After I stopped focusing on what she did to contribute to the failed marriage, I turned my energy and effort toward looking inward. I started analyzing my own shortcomings.

I learned to fight with myself.

When I learned that the divorce rate for second marriages was close to 75 percent, I felt extremely motivated to learn from my divorce because I felt terrified that if I didn't make some big changes, it was likely to happen again. I was humbled enough to want to figure out what had gone wrong, and how to avoid it in the future.

I'm not bragging here. Lord knows there have been too many times in my life when a lack of humility has got the best of me. But somewhere along the way of my own personal path, a massive mental shift happened for me, and I awakened to the reality that true humility is a sign of self-confidence, not weakness as I had always believed. I realized how my resistance to humility was a way of operating from insecurity – pretending to have it all together. I realized that being humble was an ingredient of strong men, and only weak men refused to adopt it.

Black belts in Brazilian jiu-jitsu are some of the most humble people I've met. They are supremely confident in their abilities, but simultaneously very humble. And these are some of the most seriously badass guys on the planet. If it's good enough for them, it's good enough for me.

A GREAT MARRIAGE BEGINS WITH HUMILITY

For several years, I taught a premarital class at a church every quarter. It was a fairly big class and about one hundred couples would attend every quarter. Every time I taught this class, I was intrigued by a recurring question someone in the crowd would ask nearly every quarter: "As a marriage therapist, what is the one quality or characteristic in a potential spouse you feel is essential for a happy marriage?" Since this pre-marital class was at a church, the pastors there in attendance were taken aback because my answer didn't have "Jesus" in it. But in my opinion, shared spiritual values aren't the one thing. And there's mountains of evidence to prove that. Although shared spiritual values are very important, they are not enough to keep people happily married. The most important thing is humility, which means adopting an attitude that says, "I don't know what I'm doing and I'm willing to learn". And this is what I would tell the pre-marital students every quarter. I'd say: "If you or your fiancé think you have it all figured out, please don't get married because it's likely going to end badly".

I wasn't trying to be the rainy cloud over their pre-marriage excitement, but I felt compelled to plant a seed of suspicion within them in case they realized their fiancé lacked this essential virtue. It's so important that people evaluate their future partners through this lens, and it's just as important that we keep working to grow in humility throughout the marriage journey. Without an attitude of humility, shared spiritual values don't take us very far. I've worked with too many stubborn, prideful, and arrogant hyper-spiritual couples to know that humility trumps religion.

A LACK OF HUMILITY RESULTS IN UGLY CONFLICT

When we're not as humble as we need to be, we're setting the stage for ugly conflict in our relationships. Couples that experience high levels of destructive conflict are always lacking humility. The paradigm shared by people in high conflict relationships is that the problem lies with the other person and not with themselves. That their position is right and the other position is wrong. The lack of humility creates a relationship worldview filled with accusations and finger pointing instead of humble inward looking.

We've all been there, right? You're in the middle of an argument with your wife and you're convinced that you did nothing wrong. She's crazy, and you're rational. You've got to see that there's no winning here. You know it only leads to a hopeless place filled with a lot of pain and anger. When two people are convinced the other person is wrong, they're gridlocked in a relationship stalemate.

Thankfully, with a little bravery, it's astonishing how a simple act of humility can completely put an end to an argument in seconds. A simple statement such as, "I'm open to not being right" can put the brakes on even the nastiest arguments.

That is the power of humility.

However, it's important to differentiate between being humble and being a self-deprecating, passive doormat. I'm not talking about admitting fault just to appease your angry wife or apologizing to avoid conflict. I'm talking about having enough internal strength to admit when you're wrong. True masculinity is rooted in humility, because after all, it takes significantly more power and courage to humbly identify when you're not sure, or wrong than to pretend you have it all figured out.

WITHOUT HUMILITY, WE LOSE PRECIOUS OPPORTUNITIES FOR GUIDANCE

There's so much to gain from developing humility and so much to lose by refusing to do so. When we are humble, we are also more coachable when people around us take an interest in teaching us. If we're lacking in humility, we foreclose powerful opportunities for mentorship and guidance. Which is something that we all need. No one enjoys offering help to someone who believes they have it all together. Precious opportunities to be scooped up by great mentors only come once in a while. It's a tragedy to miss such an opportunity by letting ego get in the way. A lack of humility is what keeps most men from getting relationship help. And sadly, too many men wait until the bitter end to find help, when it's usually all too late.

IMAGINE A WORLD WHERE EVERYONE SAID, "I DON'T KNOW, BUT I'M WILLING TO LEARN"

The challenge for many guys is that we're taught from an early age that we're supposed to have it all together, not need help, or to know what the hell we're doing. We're sent messages from an early age to "be the man", "take charge", or "lead by example". But when it comes to marriage, we generally don't know what we're doing. At least I didn't. But I faked it and tried for many years to pretend that I knew. It was only to my detriment. How much easier and smoother would things go in our lives if we didn't feel the need to protect our fragile egos by acting like we knew what we were doing all the time? I've learned that I can spare myself a lot of pain and that life operates so much better when I'm able to say, "I don't know!"

How would you evaluate your own level of humility as a husband? Is this something that's hard for you to do? If so, please know that you're not alone; many guys struggle with it. We're taught as little boys that being humble is a sign of weakness. But that couldn't be further from the truth. Learning to be appropriately humble when it's necessary is one of the most difficult and important aspects of becoming a Black Belt Husband. When we see how humility can transform arguments in a matter of seconds, we can begin to internalize the value of saying "I don't know what I don't know". In my experience working with men, the greatest resistance to adopting more humility comes from a fear of weakness. We fear that if we admit we don't have it all together, our spouse might take advantage of us in a moment of vulnerability.

But in reality, it rarely plays out this way. What's more likely, and what I've seen time and time again, is that your willingness to adopt humility will lead to your wife moving into the same humble posture. If being a leader in your marriage is important to you (something we will get to in a later chapter), this is what it looks like. Consider leading by example and showing your wife you're brave enough to humbly admit your relationship deficits. Cultivate a genuine ability to clearly see where things could change for you and humbly acknowledge them.

QUESTIONS TO ASSESS YOUR COURAGE WITH HUMILITY

- One common misconception about humility is that it's a sign we lack confidence. In fact, the opposite is true. True humility is a reflection of supreme confidence. Do you see humility as a sign of your confidence? Could beliefs you hold about humility keep you from cultivating more of it?
- As humans, we all have our own blind spots. These are the areas of our lives that other people may see, but we have a hard time seeing ourselves. How easy or hard is it for you to ask others to confront or kindly critique elements of your personality?
- Apologizing to simply keep the peace or to avoidantly move on from a fight is perilous. If we do this, we'll eventually feel resentment. Do you have a tendency to say "I'm sorry" from a position of passivity or conflict avoidance? It's important to see how this is not humility, but simply an avoidance strategy.
- When we have a hard time with humility, we can be defensive and unwavering with our positions. Have you ever been accused of needing to be right all the time?
- Offering a genuine apology can be very difficult if we have a hard time with humility. How easy or hard is it for you to say, "I'm sorry" and really mean it?

BLACK BELT HUSBAND TRAINING: PRACTICAL SOLUTIONS TO DEVELOP MORE HUMILITY

Before we can move forward toward higher-ranking belts, we have to get humility right. We also need to see that humility and self-deprecation are worlds apart; we can sometimes confuse these two things. We have to see humility as a cornerstone virtue of a Black Belt Husband. If humility is something that's been difficult for you, below are a few things you can do to think of it differently:

METHOD #1 – RECOGNIZE YOU'RE NOT ALONE IN THE STRUGGLE

One of the biggest obstacles to embracing humility is that we fear we are alone with our struggle. Many of us carry shame regarding the things we struggle with in relationships. As a result, we have a very hard time admitting them. Whatever your relationship struggles may be, millions of other men struggle with the same exact thing.

You are not alone, I promise you that.

And if more men were open and honest about their inner lives and the things they struggle with, then it would pave the way for other men to open up and be honest as well. If you think of yourself as a leader or role model, then commit to being more transparent with the areas of your relationship that you need to improve. You'll be better for it and you'll help other men too. It takes a lot of courage to admit you don't have it all together.

METHOD #2 – GIVE UP ON NEEDING TO BE RIGHT

A common stumbling block to humility is our need to be right. This need can show up in the most uneventful conversation or in the middle of an ugly fight. The need to be right isn't a sign of strength and mature masculinity. Instead, the need to be right is a dead giveaway of our fragility and immaturity. As long as we need to insist that we're in the right, we preclude ourselves from learning something new.

This is the antithesis of humility.

We've all been there, though. We've committed to a course of action in order to be right as opposed to learning and being open. If we want to get out of ugly power struggles, we need to give up on the need to be right. Life becomes so much more peaceful when we do it. As the cliché goes, we can be right or we can be married.

METHOD #3 – DEVELOP A NEW PERSPECTIVE OF HUMILITY

Humility is a cornerstone of mature masculinity. It's the embodiment of strength and power. True humility is not a sign of weakness nor does it make you less of a man. False pride from being insecure is a sign of weakness though, and it usually shows up as stubbornness or rigidity with beliefs. True strength looks like a willingness to admit wrongdoing, shortcomings, and deficits. We embrace humility because we recognize it as a virtue of mature masculinity and see the overwhelming positive benefits it brings to relationships.

TO GET BETTER AT CONFLICT, FOCUS ON HUMILITY AND LESS ON COMMUNICATION SKILLS

Lots of marriage help resources offer suggestions on how to limit ugly fighting or destructive conflict in marriage. Some will talk about fair fighting rules, effective communication, active listening, etc. These are not bad suggestions and they certainly have their place in improving marriages.

But truthfully, they are absolutely useless if you're not able to approach arguments with humility. Using any communication tool without a baseline level of humility will only lead to more frustration as you realize the communication tool is just serving a dug-in and entrenched position. You may begin trying harder or change directions to employ a new tool, only to realize that one doesn't work either. I've even seen the "communication tool" serve as a new weapon for an arrogant and prideful person.

Unfortunately, it will never work to apply the right solution without the right motive. Let's not waste time trying those strategies. If you're able to approach conflict in your relationship with a sense of openness, non-defensiveness, and a posture of humility that says, "I am willing to see my contribution here", the fight will end. Period. You don't have to be masterful tactician with perfect communication skills to get this right. You simply have to be a mature man, embodying some humility.

Humility can be all you need to put an abrupt stop to any argument. It can be a potent virtue that restores civility to any relationship. Conversely, applying communication tools without a posture of humility runs the risk of making the problem worse. The good news here is that you don't need to have an arsenal of tools, tricks, or right things to say. You just need to take a deep breath, and humbly own your part.

Getting stuck in the gridlock of an argument feels horrible. I've been there too; I know. It's exhausting, defeating, and can spin you into some really dark places. If you want to improve your navigation of conflict, you have to start with humility.

WHITE BELT SKILLS TEST

PRACTICAL SKILL NEEDED TO MOVE FORWARD

It takes a lot of courage and a little bit of badassness to be humble. As we develop the willingness to admit wrongdoing, errors, or areas in our relationship that need some attention, we challenge our ego, our pride, and our self-perception of feeling weak. It can feel shameful to be humble, but only if we view it through an inaccurate lens.

The irony of humility is that we display strength by acknowledging our limitations. We must remember that we all get it wrong sometimes. What's so bad about joining the human race as a non-perfect person?

Nothing.

Black Belt Husbands are always learning and expanding by virtue of adopting an attitude of humility.

Required Skill: A Meaningful Apology Rooted in Humility

One very practical method of displaying humility is in apologies. Apologies can be hard because they require a humble posture. Before we can move on to blue belt work, we need to nail the sincere apology. A good apology can be transformative.

Apologizing can get way too complicated when not done well. It needs to be simple and direct. Apologies are one of those things in life where less is more. When we apologize, we need to remember just a few things:

1. If you're really not sorry (not in a humble posture), don't say you're sorry. You end up doing more damage by saying it disingenuously than saying nothing at all.
2. But chances are, if you're really honest with yourself, you can find some aspect of a situation that calls for an apology. It just takes a little introspection to see where you erred.

3. Here are a few examples of what to say:
   a. "I am sorry I did that"
   b. "I am sorry I reacted that way"
   c. "I am sorry I hurt you like that"
   d. "I am really sorry"
   e. "I am sorry that happened again, I'm working on that"
4. Here are a few examples of what not to say:
   a. "I guess I'm sorry"
   b. "I'm sorry you took it that way"
   c. "I'm sorry you misunderstood me"

A genuine apology rests on whether or not you really feel sorry. You can't fake it. This is where humility has to play a part. No communication skill can replace your genuine humility. Don't say the words or go through the motions without really feeling it. You're better off saying nothing.

CHAPTER 3

White Belt III: Consistent; Showing Up and Doing the Work

SEEING MARRIAGE AS A VERB, NOT A NOUN

How can it be possible for any of us to achieve anything successful in life if we don't consistently show up and do the work?

Marriage is no different. Without consistent positive efforts, it's not possible to have a successful marriage. And unfortunately, this is a common pitfall for many husbands; slowly, over time, taking their foot off the gas of consistent positive effort.

They stop showing up.

After feeling defeated from too many arguments. After being distracted from other things in life. Or after believing wrongly they just don't need to work as hard. They stop doing what needs to be done.

In a perfect world, we feel motivated to do what we need to do. When we're motivated, being consistent is easy. We have all the energy and desire in the world to keep showing up. But what about when we lose our motivation? When we feel like we're not making progress in our relationship? What do we do on the days when we just don't want to show up?

Black belts in Brazilian jiu-jitsu know this principle very well. Brazilian jiu-jitsu can feel like a defeating sport at times. You can go through long periods where you feel like you're not making any progress while literally getting your ass kicked every day. But the BJJ black belt expects periods of slow progress to be part of the process. Therefore, they keep showing up to class time after time, even when they don't want to, or feel like it. Their desire to achieve their goals in BJJ is what drives their steadfast commitment to expertise and mastery.

The same goes for Black Belt Husbands. Consistency in marriage means doing the small things when no one is looking, when we don't want to do so, and when we don't get anything in return. Especially when we don't get anything in return.

We commit to consistently showing up because we've made a declaration that marriage is important to us. The refusal to show up contradicts our value system and what matters to us. We honorably continue to show up as an expression of our virtue.

When we become unmotivated, lazy, too passive, or take our partners for granted, we put our marriage at dire risk.

But being consistent in marriage is not the same as being anxious and living fearfully. We don't believe that everything will fall apart if we aren't perfect. Not at all. We simply move forward with positive momentum and understand that we must maintain an active, positive progression in marriage. When we are consistent, we live out the reality that marriage is a verb, not a noun. The mature man recognizes that greatness, in any endeavor, requires consistency regardless of whether or not he wants to.

Black Belt Husbands live out their marriages this way. They recognize marriage as a living, breathing entity that requires attention and consistent effort. Black Belt Husbands also know that the rewards far outweigh the effort. But even in times of no rewards, the effort remains.

THE KEY TO SHOWING UP: CONSISTENCY

It's easy to be consistent when your marriage is working well. You feel great and it's easier to want more of the feeling. When the relationship feels tense and unfulfilling, consistency becomes the great separator between Black Belt Husbands and all other husbands. These are the times when we need to show up the most. So, what does showing up look like? Consistently showing up can mean many things, but here are a few easy examples to get the idea:

- Being civil with your partner, even when you're angry. Or even when she's angry.
- Taking an interest in her day, even when you have a lot on your mind. Or when she's not taking an interest in your day.
- Thinking about what you can do to improve the quality of your connection with her, in ways that are important to her. Not simply in ways that are important to you.
- Honoring your obligations and commitments, which make you trustworthy with her.
- Helping out around the house, because that is important to her. Even if you feel like it's not your job.
- Not being defensive when she asks something of you, or challenges you.
- Greeting her when you see her as somebody that you care to see and not someone that you're irritated to see.
- And a thousand other things that reflect consistent positive momentum.

These are just a few examples of a myriad of different ways you can show up in your marriage. These are the little things that are not optional, and are actually required of us to make the marriage work well. These are not the big home runs, but the simple singles and doubles that can change the game dramatically over time.

Consistently showing up is living out the statement: "My marriage is very important to me". Are you living in a way that reflects your wife is supposed to be one of the most important people in your life?

But how do you consistently show up when things are getting bad, when you're not getting your needs met, or you find your wife to be horribly annoying and irritating?

During these moments, we dig deep, holding to our value system that orients our action, and committing to living out our dedication to becoming a Black Belt Husband.

Of course, during the marriage journey we're going to have periods when we feel beat down and unhappy. This is an expected part of sharing our lives with someone that we sometimes are not going to like. During these moments, we need to continue showing up and putting in the work despite our feelings. Because our desire to become great husbands, and leaving a powerful legacy trumps our temporary uncomfortable feelings.

Some guys are paralyzed by *how* to show up. They fixate so much on doing the right thing that they don't show up at all. We want to be mindful that we're showing up with positive intentionality. It's far better than not showing up at all. We don't have to always get it right, we simply have to show up with an attitude that reflects our commitment for improvement.

In BJJ, there are training days when nothing works and you get your ass kicked badly. You feel totally defeated. You start to doubt that you're really cut out for the sport and you wonder if you want to attend class the next day. BJJ black belts have felt these moments repeatedly, but they persist and push through despite their momentary waning joy for the martial art. This perseverance is how they became BJJ black belts, and it's the same perseverance and commitment to consistency that will help us reach our goal of becoming masterful husbands.

EVERYTHING WORTH HAVING TAKES EFFORT AND INTENTIONALITY

If we're going to accomplish anything worthwhile, we're going to have to put in work. In fact, we know nothing great has ever happened without a lot of hard work and dedication. Having a great marriage is the same. One of the greatest tragedies in modern marriage is the belief that a great marriage is possible without a lot of intentionality and internal motivation. For different reasons, many of us have adopted the mindset that marriage should work without the need for continual progression and positive momentum.

This passive stance is one of the biggest contributors to the demise of marriages.

Passivity becomes the cancer eroding the relationship over time. So why do people adopt such a passive stance in marriage?

The truth is that marriage takes effort and people naturally resist what is hard. We can wrongly believe or miscalculate how much effort it takes, often erring on the side of too little effort. We can commit the fatal flaw of marriage; taking each other for granted. Black Belt Husbands differ from everyday husbands in that they are continually motivated by the prospect of mastery in their role as husband and they're not afraid to put in the hard work to get there.

COMPLACENCY IS A MARRIAGE DEATH SENTENCE

When I was a kid, my dad never told me: "Quentin, here's the deal. You're about to embark on this marriage journey and I think you need to know what you're signing up for. You're choosing to be married, which is going to test you. It's going to be a lot of work. The experience will be worth it all in the end, but you need to understand that it's not easy. It will require a lot of intentionality and effort, and you'll want to give up along the way".

I wish he had said that, but he didn't know that either. Like many guys, I entered my first marriage with a completely warped understanding of what marriage was. I just thought it was a thing you did when you loved someone, a way to symbolize and crystalize your relationship. I had no idea that marriage required dedication, consistency, effort, and a great presence of mind. I thought that I could mostly coast and it would all work out. How wrong I was. I know most guys would never admit to thinking this way, but so many husbands play out their marriage like this.

When husbands stop consistently showing up or have too little of it in the first place, the outcome is a slow erosion of the marriage over time. Guaranteed.

Complacency is a marriage's death sentence. Without committing to the consistent positive action, we're destined to treat marriage as something static, instead of something that needs continual attention. Complacent husbands, often unknowing of their missteps, are accused of emotionally neglecting their partners. But in my experience working with men, the neglect is never intentional. Complacent husbands do love and care for their wives, they simply have a critical and deep misunderstanding of how relationships work and the effort necessary to sustain them.

They see their title of husband as a noun instead of a verb requiring action.

This lack of understanding among many husbands propels them into a trap of seeing their marital relationship as something that can be on cruise control. They often don't realize that they are on cruise control approaching a cliff. And so sadly, they are almost always caught off guard when their wives initiate a divorce. When they awaken from the shock, they always say, "I had no idea we were headed there". And they really mean it. These are good men without ill intent. They simply did not understand the need for consistency and positive action in their marriage.

Some men who have followed in the footsteps of their fathers, have an over-determined sense of identity as it relates to their financial contribution. They understand their role to consist in being the financial providers for their families. I applaud these men for their skills in making money and their generosity - it is truly an admirable quality. Still, marriage needs more from us and we need more from our marriages. Limiting our function as husbands to being financial providers will create a relationship of sterile cohabitants that, over time, resembles something more akin to a business partnership. Black Belt Husbands are great at being income providers and great at consistently showing up in other ways too.

Staying committed, continuing to show up, and refusing to let complacency take hold, can be challenging over the long haul, especially in times when we're not feeling motivated. Most husbands, statistically speaking, will unfortunately begin to drop off here. They will not have the understanding of the importance for consistency and stamina to continually show up and be active in their marriages. Many will divorce due to a lack of consistency, and even if they stay married, their marriage will be mostly unsatisfying. I wish that wasn't so, but the truth is being a masterful husband, moving toward Black Belt Husband is an honored achievement and it's not for everyone.

LIVING YOUR VALUES IS AUTHENTIC MASCULINITY

To reach Black Belt Husband, we have to show up consistently and be wary of complacency. Marriage requires positive action on our part and resting on our laurels is not a quality of Black Belt Husbands.

So, now that you know this, what are you going to do about it? Does reaching this goal matter enough to you? Are you going to be a man of your word, honor your commitments, and live out your vow to show up for better or for worse?

This is where the rubber meets the road, my friend.

We can proselytize all day about values and integrity, but how does it actually show up in our relationships, in real life? In the trenches. We have to ask ourselves honestly: are we actually living it out or are we simply virtue signaling to the world that we have good ideals while our lives reflect something different?

True masculinity requires that our lives be in alignment with our values. This is the definition of integrity. If we have a value system that says marriage is important to us, then we have an obligation to ourselves to live that out daily. No more complacency.

ARE YOU STILL "SHOWING UP TO CLASS"?

So where do you think you stack up on this continuum of being actively engaged or complacent in your marriage? Let's take a look at a few questions that can get you thinking about how your own relationship aligns with your value system.

I'm going to make an assumption when I ask these questions that having a good marriage is important to you. I'm going to assume that on your wedding day, you declared to yourself, your wife to be, and a whole bunch of other people that you were committed to your marriage. And I'll assume that you want to be a man of your word and honor your commitments.

- When you were first married, you were motivated to keep your relationship feeling good. Have you lost your motivation? Without blaming your wife, why?
- Being motivated in marriage means doing the small things day in and day out. It's smiling to your partner. It's saying "hello" in a kind way. It's asking them about their day. Simple, but meaningful gestures that communicate she's important to you. How would you rate yourself at consistently doing these things?

- If your marriage isn't working smoothly, how much of that is because you may have stopped showing up in your relationship with positive action?
- A relationship is like a plant you're trying to grow. It will need watering, good soil, sunlight, and continual nurturance. Are you tending to your relationship this way?
- Many men still wrongly believe that being income providers is their primary way of showing up in the marriage? How much do you see this being your primary role as a husband?
- In prior generations, it was more common for husbands to see their role as bread winner as the totality of their marriage obligation. It doesn't mean these were bad guys, it just means we had a different set of expectations in a different time. Do you feel this way of being a husband is what was role-modeled for you?
- You say marriage is important to you. That's a value you carry. Knowing that complacency is a death sentence in marriage, are you in alignment with your own value system?

BLACK BELT HUSBAND TRAINING: ADDRESSING THE MOTIVATION KILLERS

How do we stay consistently engaged in our marriage over the long haul? The answer lies in understanding the common marriage traps that can kill our success. We need to be mindful of how *impatience* and a *lack of gratitude* are obstacles to our goal of becoming Black Belt Husbands. This mindfulness will help us to continually show up in the day-to-day, even when things feel hard,

Lack of gratitude

There's nothing that kills the positive momentum in relationships faster than a lack of gratitude for our partners. Have you ever been caught in this mind trap? You know, when every little thing she does begins to irk you and you can't stop thinking about it. When you get stuck in this negative mental loop, it becomes self-reinforcing, and the negativity breeds more negativity. All of a sudden, something that seemed trivial and benign begins to look like grounds to end your marriage. When you live in this space for a prolonged period of time, you're destined to stop showing up positively in your relationship. On the way to Black Belt Husband, you have to be very careful about it. You have to recognize that a lack of gratitude can quickly be the one thing that kills your positive consistent action.

Instead of living in this lack of gratitude, mature men are able to pause and reflect on their relationship with a sense of gratitude and an ability to see goodness. This isn't living in denial, it's seeing your relationship realistically. Your relationship isn't all bad.

How often do you spend time simply reflecting on what you feel grateful for in your marriage?

In BJJ, we can see how this attitude plays such an important role. When we become less than grateful for our training partners, our teachers, or even our opportunity to be on the mat, we don't last for long. The sport is too demoralizing and challenging to be consistent unless we feel an intrinsic sense of gratitude to be able to participate in something special.

Marriage is the same. Consider starting a thirty-day gratitude list to foster more appreciation for your wife - even if you don't feel like it. It's not hard to be grateful when things are going well, but it can be very challenging to get in touch with it when you're irritated with her. When you do this, you will undoubtedly feel more optimistic about your relationship, which in turn, will boost your positive, consistent action.

Impatience

Wherever you're at in your relationship, it's important to remember that change happens slowly.

Sometimes very slowly.

People, for better or worse, can be slow to change. A relationship between two people can be even slower to change. When we're in a bad place in our marriage, it's natural to want to see change as quick as possibly. We're desperate for positive change because we don't feel good. But when we get too impatient, we can easily feel defeated and pessimistic when it's not happening as fast as we want. Then we begin to wonder if something more troubling is wrong with ourselves, our partners, or the relationship.

Impatience can lead to a certain type of hopelessness that blocks us from showing up. But if we give ourselves permission to accept that the process of change often moves slowly, we'll feel differently about it. In BJJ, impatience is probably the number one reason why people quit the sport. They want to move faster than the sport will allow and their impatience can result in walking away prematurely. BJJ black belts have been able to ride it out and make it to the end. Black Belt Husbands have the same ability to ride it out with a sense of resolved patience when things are not going well. As you develop patience, you can settle into confidence as you continue down the path of positive consistency in your marriage. Remember, we're all in this for the long haul and change happens gradually. Let's not allow a lack of patience keep us from showing up.

CONSISTENCY IS THE NECESSARY OXYGEN TO THE MARRIAGE

When we commit to showing up in marriage with consistency, it can dramatically change the overall temperature. Consistently showing up is challenging because we often let our defensiveness get in the way. When we stop consistently showing up, we're essentially resigning ourselves to failure in the marriage.

We're saying, through our actions, that we've given up.

If you're still willing to work at it, then you owe it to yourself to show back up in a consistent way.

When we communicate that we've given up through our lack of effort, we starve the relationship of air. The oxygen of every relationship is our willingness to value it enough to put in a little work that demonstrates our care. It doesn't have to be exhausting or elaborate, just a little intentionality. It might be as simple as a nice gesture, an act of kindness, or an offer to help with something. Any of it and all of it can easily turn the tide in the most strained of relationships. When your wife sees you showing up with consistent effort, she's going to feel like she really matters to you.

WHITE BELT SKILLS TEST

PRACTICAL SKILL NEEDED TO MOVE FORWARD

In order to become Black Belt Husbands, we have to move from a view of marriage as a passive endeavor to a view of marriage as an entity that needs tending to if it's to flourish. We have to see marriage as a verb, instead of a noun.

Required Skill: 30 Days of 5:1

Black Belt Husbands are very good at showing up for their wives. They see the importance of consistently working on the marriage and perfecting their craft. In fact, there is a mountain of evidence that shows the most successful husbands have a disproportionate amount of positive experiences with their wives. It's roughly five to one. Five positive interactions to every one negative interaction.

In troubled marriages, this ratio is often flipped. No one, no matter how committed they feel, can last very long with that type of prolonged negativity.

Over the next thirty days, I want you to live out this five to one ratio. I want you to be deliberate about showing up in your relationship with five positive encounters for every one negative encounter.

Even if you don't feel like it.

You only have to do thirty days as an experiment. At the end of the thirty-day period, I'm confident you will be very surprised at how different your relationship feels. What you'll see is that your wife will begin matching your five to one ratio. When you show up, it will inspire her to love you in the ways you've been seeking. This experiment is so powerful that it can end up being a total game changer. There is much wisdom in continuing to show up to do the right thing, especially when things are not working well. I don't mean sweeping things under the rug. There will be plenty of time to get to those things, but for now, I simply want you to commit to an experiment of showing up purposefully for thirty days.

Here are some examples of positive interactions to reach the five to one ratio:

- Walking through the door at the end of the day with a smile.
- Sending your wife a loving text message without expecting anything in return.
- Asking your wife if there's anything you can do to help her.
- Enthusiastically greeting your wife.
- Saying "Have a nice day, I'm going to miss you" when you leave for the day.
- Sitting down with your wife and asking her what's on her mind.
- Asking your wife to meet you for lunch out of the blue.

You get the idea. Anything that is positive counts toward the five to one ratio. Keep track of your progress by logging what you've done at the end of each day in your journal. If you can reach the five to one ratio over thirty days, you'll be the big beneficiary by what it will do for your relationship. This is Black Belt Husband work.

WHITE BELT ATTRIBUTES SUMMARY

Before we move on to blue belt, let's recap what we need to know to move forward from the fundamentals of white belt. What's really important to understand is that we must master our white belt skills because everything from this point forward is built upon our ability to be more self-aware, more humble, and more consistent.

White Belt I—Self-Awareness Summary:

The essence of self-awareness is to focus on ourselves and look inward as opposed to placing blame or focusing on our partners. As we cultivate more self-awareness, we understand that we cannot change our partners. We can only change ourselves, our thoughts and perceptions, and our reactions to scenarios where we get stuck. We realize also that our improved reactions through looking inward often creates a reciprocity of positive reactions from our partner. As we become more self-aware, we move from "fighting with our partners" to "fighting with ourselves".

White Belt II—Humility Summary:

Humility, not to be confused with self-depreciation, is an essential part of the white belt process. Humility says: "I don't have all the answers, but I'm willing to learn". Humility is a state of mind, an attitude, and a way of being in relationship. Humble people are willing to ask for help and don't pretend, out of insecurity, to have all the answers. We see that this insecurity only precludes us from getting the assistance we need. Humility as a virtue is massively attractive because it represents deep, and authentic strength - something all women crave.

White Belt III—Consistency Summary:

Consistently showing up is the lifeblood of relationships. It's the oxygen that keeps the relationship going and prevents it from dying a slow death. When we stop showing up, we're communicating to our partners through action that we are resigning. There's no faster way to kill goodness in a marriage than to stop consistently showing up. Showing up doesn't require a ton of effort, it just requires some positive intentionality, good will and a recognition of its necessity. The rewards far outweigh any effort.

Congratulations!
You've graduated from White Belt!

SECTION TWO

The Blue Belt Journey; Developing Self-Confidence and Strength

Jiu-jitsu does not build character, it reveals it. We are all born with immeasurable courage and determination, it is as we go through the trials of rigorous training that we discover those gifts.
—Ricardo Almeida, BJJ Black Belt and UFC fighter

WELCOME TO BLUE BELT

The blue belt journey is an exhilarating part of the road toward Black Belt Husband. The blue belt training will crystalize our in-born strengths and we'll learn new ways of relating that expand our self-confidence. As blue belts, we'll face adversity and overcome fears that keep us from having a more rewarding relationship. In white belt work, we mastered some important fundamentals which will now allow us to take greater risks.

Risks that require courage. Our own sense of comfort will be challenged as we step into new horizons of being a husband. The blue belt journey, when complete, deepens our self-confidence as we realize the power in our healthy masculinity.

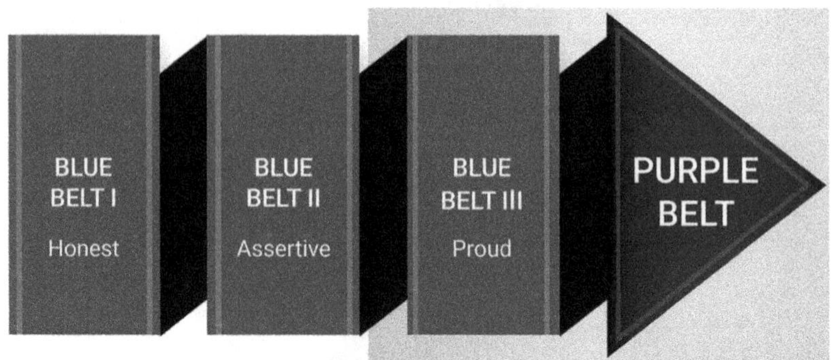

BLUE BELT WORK

CHAPTER 4

Blue Belt I: Honest; Being Truthful with Ourselves and Others

HONESTY IS THE BEDROCK OF ANY GREAT RELATIONSHIP

The blue belt journey begins with our need to evaluate the level of honesty in our lives and in our marriages. The blue belt journey demands that we take an honest look at our relationship on all levels and how we feel about it. Even in the face of conflict. Too often, men fall victim to the trappings of being too passive, deferential, or acquiescent in relationships out of fear of conflict. Adopting the "happy wife, happy life" mindset to their detriment. Being deferential is a wonderful attribute when we're operating from strength, but for many men the difficulty lies with being deferential due to their fear that it may provoke conflict.

When this happens, we become imprisoned by our passivity.

Hating ourselves for getting walked on and resenting our partners horribly.

The negative consequences of not being honest are innumerable. But before we can be honest with our partners, we have to be open and honest with ourselves about what really matters to us. This kind of honesty requires a solid sense of clarity about what we really want and why we want it.

In blue belt work we realize that a great marriage is not possible without lots of honesty and with increased honesty usually comes increased conflict. Great relationships are not conflict free. In fact, any great relationship rests on a foundation of honesty, which simultaneously rests on a foundation of managing conflict well. When we can operate this way, instead of shying away from honesty or natural conflict, we're on our way to Black Belt Husband.

KEEPING THE PEACE WILL LEAD TO AN EMOTIONAL PRISON SENTENCE

When you're not honest in your marriage you may be able to fake it for some length of time, but the relationship will eventually implode under the pressure of growing resentments and denied longings.

As a kid growing up in a high-conflict home, I developed a serious aversion to conflict from an early age. I saw conflict handled so poorly that I wanted nothing of it. So instead of being honest, I would care-take and people-please as much as I could as a way to avoid conflict. I did this until I eventually would blow up with fits of anger. It took me some time to figure out that I could be honest about what I wanted without dominating others or acquiescing to them. Being honest and tolerating the reactions of others has been a work in progress for me and it's something I'm mindful of often, even today. When we get better at doing this a whole new world of freedom opens up. You can speak your mind freely even in the face of adversity.

Being honest often means declaring that our needs and wants are important to us. When we forgo these declarations for the sake of keeping the peace, our relationships often begin a downward slide into passive aggressive resentment. Our intention, when we're honest, is never to be hurtful to anyone, but we realize that others might be hurt along the way and that's just part of life. We don't approach honesty as bullies demanding that others meet our needs or give in to our tyrannical demands. That's what children do. We're talking about being mature enough to know what we want, and to speak our truths about it. And we realize that sometimes the natural consequence of being honest in relationships is that people get hurt. All the same, we're nearly guaranteed that we will always hurt ourselves if we're dishonest or denying what's important to us.

Why is it so challenging for men to be honest in marriage? Married men in the twenty-first century have been molded since early childhood to be passive and deferential in their relationships. We've been taught that being "nice" and sacrificial is the better way. Infidelity rates, addiction statistics, and depression rates among men tell us this strategy isn't working. This part of the Black Belt Husband journey is about waking up to the reality that our tendency to be nice as a means to keep the peace is destroying our souls and killing our relationships.

Whenever two people are open and honest in a relationship, they bring forward their competing needs and wants, and everything gets set on the table for an open conversation. When these needs diverge, conflict may arise. But we can't be afraid of conflict when it comes from a place of healthy self-assertion. Openly and honestly sharing our wants and needs, even if they're at odds with the wants and needs of our partners, is an essential ingredient for healthy relationships. We need to tell the truth about what's important to us because it's how our partners get to know us, wholly and completely. We get to show them the good, the bad, and the ugly. They might not always like what they learn, but that's part of the deal in marriage. If we deny ourselves through dishonesty or omission, we will become resentful and disconnected. Self-denial is the poison pill for many marriages.

WITHOUT HONESTY, WE'RE LIVING AN UNSUSTAINABLE LIE

When we're not honest, we're essentially pretending to be somebody that we're not. The easiest way to be dishonest is through lying by omission and denying what's important or pretending that it's not important. This is the classic setup for the cliché mid-life crisis. The guy turns fifty, gets a Maserati, and leaves his wife for someone twenty years younger. This cliché mid-life crisis story is always a result of denied longings. I've worked with a hundred of these types of guys and the realization is always the same when the dust settles. They all wish they had been more honest about what was important to them. Black Belt Husbands don't have mid-life crises because they're not suffocating under 25 years of denied longings.

You see, there's a little paradox at play. Our wives, partly, want us to be compliant so they can get what they want from us. That's human nature and we can't blame them for wanting our compliance. But many wives also feel hopelessly disconnected in their marriages because their men are shells of themselves. The husband's compliance breeds the wife's loneliness. Relationships can't survive with these circumstances. The way out is to be more honest in our relationships and with ourselves. Conflict from honesty always trumps compliance that breeds disconnection.

FEMINISM AND THE SUBORDINATION OF THE MASCULINE

Many men have a hard time being honest in their marriages because they are afraid of their wives' angry reaction when they begin opening up about who they really are and what is important to them. Many men would never admit this because it's not very "manly" to be intimidated by your wife, but their passive and acquiescent behaviors tell a different story. Out of fairness to some of these guys, a lot of women are horribly cruel and mean to their husbands - that's a fact. I've worked with many. But we're not concerning ourselves here with the behavior of unhealthy women; we're here to look at how we, as men, can do something different.

Without going into a long sociological history of marriages, here is what's happened over the past few generations. Men of previous generations (think 1940's and 1950's) were typically the more dominant partner in marriages because it was culturally acceptable. But many men in this era abused their power as husbands and mistreated their wives. In response to the abusive role many husbands held, the Feminist movement was born in the 1960's, partly to claim women's rights in the context of the marriage relationship. Over the next several decades, a powerful cultural shift took place where men became more passive and compliant in marriages because it was not acceptable for them to be domineering. The Feminist movement was very important, culturally needed, and much good came from it.

But like many movements, the pendulum swung too far. Men were culturally convinced that their power as a man was destructive and what it meant to be a good husband was essentially to be a total pushover. Men stopped fighting for what was important to them and lost their masculine strength in the process. This is not a political commentary, but a quick glimpse at what has happened to men and their roles in marriage in the past few decades and why it's such a mess today. The passivity of the modern husband is killing the modern marriage because no marriage can survive with such lopsided power dynamics. Black Belt Husbands are comfortable with their power and honesty in relationships. And comfortable with their wife's power and honesty. Our need to reclaim our honesty and a certain level of comfort with conflict that comes from honesty is an essential part of our masculine health.

WHAT HAVE YOU DENIED OR BEEN DISHONEST ABOUT?

How often are you dishonest with your wife about what's really important to you? How much do you lie to yourself by denying your dreams and ambitions? Becoming a Black Belt Husband is about having an incredible marriage even in the face of adversity and conflict. Yes, these two are possible in tandem. Your relationship needs your honesty and your willingness to be true to yourself. So, what are you denying in order to keep the peace? I want you to analyze your own level of honestly using the questions below.

- What kinds of things do you enjoy doing that you've stopped doing because you fear that your wife would be disappointed?
- What aspects of your sex life are you discontent with, but you've stopped speaking up about?
- Who are the friends you've stopped engaging because you fear it will upset your relationship with your wife?
- What kinds of things do you find yourself leaving out of important conversations with your wife for fear of rocking the boat?
- What hobbies, interests, and adventures have you stopped dreaming about because you think good married men don't do things like that?
- What is one thing that absolutely drives you insane about your wife, but you've given up telling her?
- What kinds of resentments do you have toward your wife that you've chosen to ignore, not out of compassion but out of fear?

WE DON'T NEED A MASSIVE OVERHAUL - WE JUST NEED A NEW DIRECTION

Again, honesty is not about purposely hurting people. All the same, if people get hurt when we're honest, so be it. It's important that we be mindful about how we deliver the message and interact with others, but we can't let the fear of hurting others, or others getting angry, prevent us from speaking truthfully in relationships. A good relationship is not possible without deep levels of honesty.

The journey is to become supremely honest in your relationships, but we first have to recognize that our fear of conflict holds us back. . Until we get more comfortable with conflict, we'll always default back to being dishonest, lying by omission, and denying what's important to us.

The process starts with looking inward and acknowledging all the ways you've been deluding yourself by pretending that important things weren't important. Part two in the process is taking baby step risks toward honesty with your wife. These are the defining moments; taking little risks of honesty when it would just be easier not to. You might be tempted to read this chapter and become overwhelmed with the thought that you need to have a massive and abrupt self-disclosure session with your wife. That's not the point. We're moving slowly and methodically. At this point, you simply want to commit to moving in a more transparent and honest direction about what matters to you.

BLACK BELT HUSBAND TRAINING: RECLAIM WHAT YOU'VE GIVEN UP

I worked with a client who used to fly planes before he got married. After he got married, his wife expressed her dissatisfaction with it. As a result, he decided to resign his pilot's license. He later realized it was the biggest mistake he made in his marriage because he set a precedent that he would deny himself in order to prevent conflict with his wife. He loved flying - it was his passion - and he regretted giving something up that he loved so dearly. Deep down, he carried a mountain of resentment toward his wife for "making him stop flying". But she didn't make him. She didn't hold a gun to his head and tell him he couldn't do it. She simply didn't like that he flew and she was entitled to her feelings about it. It wasn't her, it was his inability to tolerate conflict that was the reason he stopped flying. He lied to himself for many years and tried to convince himself that good husbands shouldn't do risky activities like fly or have interests and hobbies that wives don't like. He also believed that good husbands should care about their wives' feelings and do everything possible to accommodate them.

As we worked together, he learned the difference between being deferential out of fear and being deferential out of care. Being deferential and accommodating to our wives is fine, but we never want to do it out of fear of conflict. After addressing his fear of conflict, he eventually returned to flying. His wife was naturally disappointed and expressed her frustration about it. I told him to remain firm and commit to his love of flying even in the face of her anger. Long story short, he's flying and his wife has grown to accept it. It didn't come without some choppy waters, but in the end it was a critical move for him to reclaim a lost part of himself and learn how to assert himself in his marriage.

Now what about you? What kind of things have you given up because you thought that's what good husbands do or don't do? Being a great husband does not mean being molded into the person your wife wants you to be. Being a great husband means learning to accept and be honest with yourself. It's fine and good to acquiesce if you choose to at times, but never out of fear.

Right now, I want you to dig deep and think about one thing that you've given up or one thing that you pushed aside because you thought it wasn't worth the fight. It's the one thing that contributes to your resentment. I'm wanting you to see that the resentment is poisonous to your relationship. I want you to recommit to that one thing - no matter what. The work of Black Belt Husbands is to learn to face adversity and tolerate conflict. There's a good chance that your wife won't like what this thing is, but commit to it anyway and try to live with the discomfort that will come from the conflict.

HONESTY IS THE PATHWAY TO SELF-RESPECT AND HER RESPECT

When we become more honest in our relationships, we afford ourselves the opportunity to reclaim our happiness again. We avert the mid-life crisis out of a willingness to be honest. Honesty tends to evoke conflict, but the conflict doesn't have to be destructive or something so intolerable that we run from it. We are realizing that our job is not to spare others from hurt feelings by being dishonest. We can care about other's feelings, empathize with them, and remain steadfast in our commitment to be ruthlessly honest.

Being honest also makes you intriguing again. When you make your declarations to the world about what you want and what you're about, you become attractive to the people around you - even if they have competing needs. It's interesting that someone may have hurt feelings in response to your honesty, but they will find you more attractive at the same time.

When we're at our most honest, our wives feel less alone in the world because they know us, who we are, and connect to us at a deeper level. And feeling more connected is something that every wife deeply desires.

Being committed to a path of honesty is also the way to earn respect from your wife and to begin respecting yourself again. Many men have low levels of self-respect, even as they crave respect from their wives. If you want to earn your wife's respect, start by being honest with her. She may not like everything you have to say, but she will respect you for showing up as a strong and powerful man by being honest.

BLUE BELT SKILLS TEST

PRACTICAL SKILL NEEDED TO MOVE FORWARD

Our resentments are a road map to the places where we haven't been as honest as we needed to be. We inevitably feel resentful about things we neglect to speak up about. These places of resentment can be great teachers and we should begin to pay attention to them. I want you to create a list of all of your resentments, no matter how big or small. Once you have your list, I want you to pick three of the most important ones and share them with your wife. When you share them, your only objective is to help her understand you better. She doesn't have to like what you share. She doesn't have to agree with you. She doesn't have to change what she's doing. She might even get irritated with you for sharing them. All of that is perfectly fine. Our goal for this exercise is to simply begin the process of opening up and being more comfortable with being honest about the things that are important to you. That's it. At this point, you don't need to change anything. You don't have to expect anything to be different. You just want to begin acknowledging the resentment. This is the beginning of a new path toward transparency, honesty, and self-assertion. All essential Black Belt Husband ingredients.

CHAPTER 5

Blue Belt II: Assertive; Killing the Inner People Pleaser

MOVING FROM SIMPLY BEING HONEST TO BEING INVOLVED

In Chapter Four, we explored the importance of complete honesty even in the face of conflict. In Chapter Five, we're going to expand our definition of honesty to include being more assertive; think of it as the result of taking honesty into action.

Assertiveness is an active state. Before you can grow in assertiveness and become a more active participant in your marriage, you have to gain clarity on what you actually want and what you actually believe is important to you.

As we grow in assertiveness, we will kill the inner people pleaser that insists on making sure other people are happy, even at the expense of our own emotional health. As we become more assertive, we also refuse to get stuck in a passive or passive-aggressive role. We speak up for what we want and take responsibility for our own lives. As we grow in assertiveness, we move from the state of mind that says, "I don't care, whatever you want", to "This is what I want".

Becoming more assertive is about coming to the table of life, welcoming yourself, and joining the party to which you've been rightfully invited.

GETTING IN THE GAME OF THE RELATIONSHIP

Assertiveness is a necessary attribute for any quality relationship because without it, relationships will die a slow death of being lifeless, feeling stale and likely boring. Assertiveness supplies our wives with the necessary feeling of being partnered in marriage and when we're not assertive, the relationship feels as though it's without one of the two people. When we're not assertive, we run the risk of feeling as though the marriage is a party of one rather than two coming together as one. Black Belt Husbands recognize that assertiveness is the only way to get our needs met. Assertiveness is the healthy middle ground where we can make declarations about what is important to us, confidently.

Assertiveness keeps us on good footing and away from adopting a too passive role or a passive-aggressive role as husbands. Assertiveness is the hedge against these two undermining ways of being in marriage that are all too common for the modern husband. Black Belt Husbands see that both of these options, over time, become poisonous to the marriage and will erode any goodness in the relationship. Too many men have adopted a belief that being passive is a more 'holy' way in marriage because of the self-denial and sacrifice it requires. Only to realize that they carry mountains of resentments that inevitably bleed into the relationship in the form of passive-aggressive behavior. When passive men are honest with themselves, they see that their sacrifice is rarely made out of true sacrificial giving, but more often, it is done as a way to appease their partner and avoid the likely conflict that may come from being assertive. True sacrifice is only done out of strength, and never out of fear of conflict.

Passivity in marriage is like being in the backseat instead of grabbing the steering wheel of life and driving. When we become more assertive, our partners will begin to take more of an interest in us. Our self-confidence begins to shine through. When it comes to the theory of human attractiveness, the number one trait that attracts humans to other humans is not good looks, not money, and certainly not passivity; it's self-confidence. Assertiveness is the bedrock of self-confidence. When we're not assertive, we are prone to self-loathing for not standing up for ourselves and resentment toward our wives because we feel we have lost ourselves.

People who struggle with assertiveness often express their anger and resentment in the form of passive-aggressive behavior. For example, you're angry, but you lack the ability to simply say, "that makes me angry". Instead you communicate your anger indirectly by being undermining, sarcastic, inattentive, etc. Assertiveness eliminates all passive aggressiveness and invites you to show up in the relationship with a confident declaration about what you want and what you don't want. You know how to say "yes!", and you know how to say "no!".

The more we get comfortable with being assertive, the more it increases our self-confidence and our attractiveness. Without assertiveness, we risk becoming passive observers, or resentful, sidelined spectators. Instead, we want to adopt a mindset that forces us right into the middle of the game in marriage.

INAPPROPRIATE BLOW-UPS AND CHINESE WATER TORTURE

Have you ever been accused of blowing up at your wife or getting overly enraged about a situation that didn't seem to warrant such a strong reaction? That's what happens when we adopt too passive a role in our marriages and neglect the need to be assertive. Blowups are almost always a product of neglecting ourselves until we reach a breaking point and explode. We feel backed into a corner by our partners and explode to get their attention. But the truth is that we back ourselves into corners with passive behavior and an unwillingness to speak up for ourselves. As much as we may want to blame our wives for feeling backed into a corner, it's important to see that we place ourselves there. Thankfully, we can also take ourselves out of that position.

As we discussed in Chapter Four, our avoidance of conflict is the heart of the reason that we don't speak up enough. The rage episodes that inevitably ensue wreak havoc on our relationships. The only thing anyone remembers in the aftermath of such angry outbursts is the inappropriate, angry response. We end up losing all our credibility. It's essential that we recognize assertiveness as the way to halt these types of angry explosions. Be assertive every day, even with the small things. Without the consistency of assertive actions, we're destined for another perilous, destructive outburst. We'll be condemned that we need anger management and sent away. Being assertive changes all of that.

In addition to these emotionally disproportionate rage episodes, the other common alternative when dealing with anger is to become passive aggressive. Being passive aggressive may seem like a better alternative than the angry outbursts, but it will be just as destructive to the marriage. Passive aggressiveness is the go-to coping method for many modern husbands faced with anger.

When you're not assertive in your marriage, you will feel resentful because it will feel like you're in a one-down position. And for the non-assertive husband, this anger and resentment comes out in a cancerous passive-aggressive form. The reason passive-aggressiveness is so destructive is because it leaves the person on the receiving end feeling confused, crazy, and without a sense of equilibrium. Have you ever interacted with someone who was angry with you, even as they tried to convince you that everything was fine? It's maddening, because they take digs at your character, slight your personality, ignore you, and often hurt you with a joke, but simultaneously tell you how much they "love you". Passive-aggressive people go through all this trouble to communicate that they are mad at you instead of simply saying, "I'm mad at you". Being in a relationship with someone who's passive-aggressive feels like dying a slow, psychotic death by Chinese water torture. There's no other way around it, passive-aggressive behavior will undermine any sense of connection in relationship. So here are our options: Being aggressive is not going to work. Being passive is not going to work. Being passive aggressive is not going to work. Assertiveness is the only thing that works.

ASSERTIVENESS IS A CORNERSTONE ALPHA QUALITY

Guys, do you want to know a secret? Women love men who take charge. It's true today as much as it's been true for thousands of years. Women are wired to look for alpha qualities in potential mates because it has historically and evolutionarily represented safety for women. Despite our modern civilization and advancing technologies, we can't undo 200,000 years of evolutionary biology. Authentic masculinity doesn't shy away from claiming the role of an assertive, alpha male who takes charge. When we resort to being fear-based people pleasers, we're distorting what is good, true, and evolutionarily appropriate. Healthy masculinity cringes at fearful passivity or passive-aggressive behavior because it goes against the grain of everything in our DNA. We are wired to be assertive.

Being assertive in your relationship, and in life in general, is a cornerstone alpha quality. But people get the alpha male concept confused so it gets a bad rap in the media today. Being alpha doesn't mean being a bully or steamrolling your mate because you're a domineering asshole. In fact, you can't be truly alpha until you're humble (refer back to white belt work if you feel confused about this). The true alpha is assertive. You stand up for your beliefs, refusing to let fear keep you stifled, and you develop enough self-confidence that you can say yes to what you want, and no to what you don't want. This assertiveness is deeply masculine and craved by women. It requires self-confidence and it requires that we take risks in speaking up for ourselves. Women want their men to take charge in an assertive manner, which is not to be confused with aggression or domination. When you act assertively, and layer it on top of humility, a white belt prerequisite, your wife will begin to fall in love with you again.

ARE YOU PASSIVE, PASSIVE AGGRESSIVE, OR ASSERTIVE?

Acting in an assertive manner can be challenging for some because they don't want to be perceived as domineering bullies. Assertiveness can be easily confused with aggressiveness, but they are worlds apart. We can be massively assertive, and still kind and loving. For some guys, acting assertively can result in being called selfish or narcissistic, so they decide that it's easier to acquiesce. The degree to which husbands have the capacity to act assertively is often a reflection of their levels of self-confidence and self-assuredness. This is the work of blue belts on their way to the Black Belt Husband. Spend a little time asking yourself a few of the following questions. Let them serve as a barometer for your level of assertiveness:

- Non-assertive guys are always the ones who adopt "happy wife, happy life". Have you fallen victim to believing this cliché was the way to a good marriage?
- Do you have a hard time expressing your frustration with your wife in a direct and assertive way when your wife acts inappropriately?
- Have you limited the amount of time you spend with friends because you fear your wife's frustration about being gone too much?

- Does your wife express frustration that you never know what you want when faced with certain choices?
- Have you ever been accused of being passive aggressive as a way of communicating your anger?
- Can you recognize the times that you defer to the needs of your wife because you want to avoid conflict, but you tell yourself it's because you're just being nice?
- If you're frustrated about something, how hard or easy is it for you to simply say, "I am angry".
- You're at the grocery store to buy ice cream. You only have enough money for one flavor. You want vanilla and your wife wants chocolate. Who wins 80 percent of the time?

BLACK BELT HUSBAND TRAINING: QUIT TAKING CARE OF EVERYONE ELSE, AND START TAKING CARE OF YOURSELF

It's important to remember that being deferential is not a bad thing. In fact, it's often a wonderful quality of humanity that is a reflection of kindness and genuine care. But in our blue belt work, it's important that we spend time clarifying the why behind our deference. It's too easy to chalk up all of our deferential behavior to kindness and genuine care. That would let us off the hook without examining other possibilities. We need to consider when being deferential is a reflection of fear-based people pleasing. When we lead with passivity, it will always give rise to negative consequences over time. It's only a matter of time before we feel so stifled and backed into a corner that we emotionally explode. The good news, however, is that we can develop greater assertiveness by taking small steps in our lives to move the needle from passive behavior to assertiveness. Like all change in our lives, it may feel a little uncomfortable at first to operate more assertively, but over time and with practice it becomes something that is simply natural and spontaneous.

Before we can start acting more assertively in our relationships, we have to become clear on what's really important to us. This is something that I was so lost with for many years. If someone asked me in my twenties what was important to me, I wouldn't even know what they were talking about, let alone have an answer. Boys in our culture are rarely encouraged to get in touch with their needs. I know I wasn't.

When husbands awaken to what's important to them after years of self-denial, there can be a tendency to flip the table on their spouse. Everything becomes an assertiveness-hill-to-die-on. They can become unwavering and uncompromising about nearly everything because they confuse assertiveness with stubbornness. It's like having not eaten in a week and walking into a candy store to binge on Skittles. It won't be good for you. I want you to take it slow. To do so, I want you to begin thinking about what I call your personal non-negotiables. Your personal non-negotiables are the things in your life that really matter to you. These are the things that you need for yourself in order to live a fulfilled life. They are your must-haves. So as to not get too overwhelmed, let's start with a list of the top five personal non-negotiables that you're unwilling to compromise on any longer. These are five things in your life that you will no longer be passive about and can commit to implementing right now. Here are a few places where personal non-negotiables may need to be addressed:

- Do you have any personal non-negotiables about how you spend your free time?
- Do you have any personal non-negotiables about what foods you eat?
- Do you have any personal non-negotiables about your hobbies?
- Do you have any personal non-negotiables about how you spend money?

- Do you have any personal non-negotiables about your relationships with your friends?
- Do you have any personal non-negotiables about the way you're treated in your relationship?

When you think about your personal non-negotiables, it's important to remember that the reason you're doing it is to keep yourself from lapsing into self-hatred for being a people pleasing, fear-based accommodator, or from inevitably exploding into rage from resentments. Your personal non-negotiables keep your soul alive and keeping your soul alive matters more than anything else. I hope you don't read this as dramatic. You can't live a fulfilled life if you don't do the things that really matter to you. When you think about your personal non-negotiables, you're taking care of yourself - something that many husbands don't do very well, because we're taught from a very young age to "be strong", "be brave" and be the accommodating rescuer of others. You may be really good at taking care of everyone else while putting yourself last on the list. Create your list of personal non-negotiables and begin living them out right now. You don't need to announce them to your wife, you simply need to start living them out. Know that conflict will arise and your inner people pleaser will want to give in. Don't let it win.

FREEDOM, HAPPINESS, AND A BETTER RELATIONSHIP AWAIT YOU

When we begin acting more assertively in relationships, a whole new world of freedom begins to open up for us. We realize that we actually are the masters of our own destinies. In our assertiveness, we're no longer subjected to the whims of what others want from us. Instead, we do what we want to do and with that posture of assertiveness we begin taking responsibility for our own happiness. And we can do this while maintaining the most loving posture toward our spouse.

When we act more assertively, we come to the realization that it's up to us to advocate for our own lives. When we grow in assertiveness, we kill the inner people pleaser that obsesses relentlessly about making others happy (at our expense) and we begin to put that energy toward making ourselves happy. Developing more assertiveness always results in an increased sense of autonomy and mastery, which helps us feel more self-confident.

When we commit to assertiveness, we always reserve the right to be deferential, but not because we feel we must. Assertiveness is directly correlated with a deepening of connection. Women love men who are self-confident and when paired with the humility from white belt work, we can be sure we're on the way to becoming irresistible Black Belt Husbands.

The road toward Black Belt Husband is not easy. Similar to becoming a black belt in Brazilian jiu-jitsu, it requires doing the hard things day after day. In BJJ, less than 1 percent of the people who start as white belts ever make it to black belt. The commitment and dedication make it an achievement very few will ever reach. Reaching Black Belt Husband requires a similar level of commitment and dedication which can be challenging. Black Belt Husbands do the hard things not because they're masochistic, but because they're aiming for an achievement that makes the hard work worthwhile. Being more assertive in your relationship may not come easily. It may raise your own anxiety because you know conflict is the natural byproduct. But it's important that you move forward regardless. You can't skip this step if you want to become a Black Belt Husband.

BLUE BELT SKILLS TEST

PRACTICAL SKILL NEEDED TO MOVE FORWARD

Higher ranking belts are going to require us to get our anger in check and get more comfortable with asserting ourselves. When we act passively in our relationships out of fear, we will inevitably get angry and though we're largely angry at ourselves, we'll direct this anger toward our partners. Passive husbands work hard to suppress their angry feelings and the result is usually that they eventually explode with toxic rage. It may not happen frequently, but it's only a matter of time until the next explosion comes. These rage episodes, even if infrequent, are always eroding to the marriage. They destroy the connection we have with our partners as well as our credibility as safe and trustworthy husbands. Black Belt Husbands don't encounter these rage episodes because they've learned to be consistently assertive about what really matters to them.

Required Skill: Understanding Your Primary Emotions

In order for us to move forward toward Black Belt Husbands, we too have to find healthier expressions for our frustrations. The best way to start this process is to learn the difference between primary and secondary emotions. Primary emotions are the underlying feelings that lead to anger; anger is a secondary emotion. Anger is called secondary because it always arises in response to a more primary emotion.

Men sometimes feel weak or unmanly when they acknowledge their primary emotions. Some common examples are sadness, rejection, loneliness, overwhelm, fear, suffocation, or shame for not being good enough. When we suppress these emotions out of fear of looking weak, we are left with the alternative to become angry. Anger, is a self-protective emotion that serves as a way to insulate us from hurt. Without a better understanding of our primary emotions, we will always be one-trick ponies with anger as our go-to response for any painful experience. In order for us to move on to purple belt, we have to get a better handle on the inevitable blow-ups by becoming more aware of primary emotions. Spend some time and think about this idea. What is the primary emotion that you suppress with your anger, typically? Our job at this point is to get more clarity about our primary emotions. The more we understand them, the more we can communicate them, which will put an end to our toxic rage episodes.

Understanding the concept of primary emotions versus secondary emotions was one of the biggest aha moments I have ever experienced in my understanding of relationships. This one concept is absolutely transformative.

CHAPTER 6

Blue Belt III: Proud; Gaining Her Respect Through Self Respect

PRIDE IN OURSELVES GOES BELOW THE SURFACE

As we near the end of our blue belt journey, we begin to hold ourselves with greater confidence and a renewed sense of pride.

Rightfully so.

By this point in the journey we have worked hard. Without being arrogant, we can take pride in the work we've accomplished and the courage we've mustered to push through some difficult things. We're now going to take a look at pride and why it's necessary for Black Belt Husbands.

The kind of pride I'm referring to reflects a higher order of self-esteem and self -respect. I'm not talking about the kind of pride that is rooted in arrogance and lacks humility. Remember,

Black Belt Husband is a developmental process wherein each phase builds on the foundation laid by previous phases. The pride we're discussing rests on top of the required humility we discussed in the white belt training. When we combine a healthy sense of pride with humility, we become irresistible husbands. To paint a picture in your mind of the type of pride I'm talking about, let me begin with a story.

A few years ago, I worked with Jason and Sara in couples counseling. We discovered that the communication problems they brought forward as their reason for needing counseling were not the root of their problems. A few months into counseling, Sara revealed she'd been having an affair with a co-worker. Of course, Jason was devastated. We spent about a year repairing the damage wrought by the affair and explored the problems that brought it about.

Infidelity is a complicated issue in couples counseling. All couples therapists understand that an affair is most often simply a symptom of a deeper underlying problem in the relationship. The job of the couples counselor is to get to the root causes behind the affair. As we worked through the reality of the affair together, we discovered a variety of contributing factors on both sides of the relationship. These factors included ugly arguments, dishonesty, and a growing sense of disconnection. These factors accumulated over time to such a point that the couple grew apart in a catastrophic way. Of course, none of these things justify an affair, however, when we look at affairs in terms of underlying relationship patterns, we stand before something that looks less like a moral problem and more like a set of dynamics informing the health of the relationship. Sara did a good job of owning her bad decision and ultimately took responsibility for her choices. She felt terrible and was filled with guilt for what she had done. She was raised in a virtuous family and infidelity wasn't something she identified as a part of her world. She felt very sad and ashamed for how she hurt her husband. Over time, Jason was also able to see how his action and inaction contributed to the affair. No, he didn't step out on the marriage, but he wasn't exactly innocent in the bigger story.

When Jason and Sara met, he was a soldier in the U.S. Marine Corps. He was youthful, vibrant, athletic, and full of life. But something interesting happened in their first year of marriage. Sara recalled it with great detail.

He let himself go. He stopped caring about his weight or keeping himself groomed. When he came to my office, he hadn't seen the inside of a gym in over five years. On the other hand, Sara made a point of continually putting her best foot forward in the relationship. She recounted times when she would get changed into something sexier before Jason got home from work in an attempt to be attractive to him. When they originally showed up to my office, I remember noticing the discrepancy between how the two looked. Jason had a five-day disheveled beard, was forty pounds overweight, and wore distastefully baggy clothes to compensate for his poor body image. Sara, on the other hand, was immaculate. She wore form-fitting, fashionable clothes, attractive makeup and had an incredible figure for someone who'd given birth to a second child only a year earlier.

As Sara's shame and guilt subsided, she sheepishly hinted at her dissatisfaction with how Jason took care of himself. She was very reluctant to say anything about it because she didn't want to hurt his feelings. As I pressed her to be more open and honest, she began letting us know why it really mattered to her. In moments of tearful expression, she told Jason how his neglect for himself made her feel unimportant.

She had come to believe Jason no longer cared about her.

She felt that Jason's unwillingness to take pride in himself was a sign that he had given up on her and the relationship. When it continued for years, she eventually became interested in another man who showed her a minimal level of attentiveness. By no means am I absolving Sara of responsibility for making poor decisions. She has to live with the guilt and remorse that she caused herself and her family. However, I've seen the pattern too many times to know that it could happen to any one of us. If we stop caring about how we carry ourselves, what message does this send to our partners? Are we communicating to them that they are cherished? Of course not. Instead, we're communicating to them that we don't really care. That we're taking them for granted.

OUR MARRIAGE STILL DESERVES OUR DIGNITY

When we first started dating our partners, we were very mindful of taking care of ourselves. We obsessed about which shirts looked best on us. We cared because we knew the relationship hinged to some degree on this level of care. And in the beginning, we would often go out of our way to make sure we got it right. We tried hard because it was our way of showing that we really cared. Why then, do we stop thinking this way when we get married and have a few years under our belt? Well, the truth is that we stop because we're lazy and take our partners for granted. If you're honest with yourself, you'll agree. It may sound harsh, but it's true.

Perhaps some of you reading this might be thinking, "but isn't it superficial to think this way?", or "I want a relationship that is more meaningful and doesn't revolve around my appearance". To that I would say, you're living in a fantasy. If you're really honest with yourself, you expect the same of your wife. Taking pride in yourself and being an impressive husband is much deeper than the actual practicalities of looking good. Putting effort into yourself communicates a very powerful message to your wife.

It tells her one thing: "You are important enough that I continually want to impress you".

Putting effort into yourself also communicates that you value yourself as well. This is not shallow or about superficial vanity. Taking pride in yourself communicates something much more powerful. The way you carry yourself matters very much to your spouse, and you have to get it right as a Black Belt Husband. When you carry yourself with self-respect, it also earns her respect.

WE SHOULD CARE *WHILE* BEING MARRIED

Have you ever met someone who was newly divorced and post-marriage they completely transform their physical appearance? When people do these post-marriage makeovers, the message they are sending to the world is: "My husband/wife was not important enough to me to have pride and self-respect, but now that I've lost them I will begin to do so". To be honest, I was that guy. I took my relationship for granted and didn't think that maintaining my physical presence mattered much. I would never have admitted this to anyone, but I lived with the idea that I was married now and could afford to care a little less.

How unfortunate for anyone who has to go through divorce to see the relevance and importance of maintaining pride and self-respect in marriage. Can we learn that we have a need for healthy pride and self-respect before we reach divorce? I think we can, if we awaken to the deeper messages we communicate to our spouse when we stop taking care of ourselves.

When we stop taking care of ourselves, we risk becoming unappealing to our partners. Ask yourself: Would you be attracted to somebody who has stopped taking care of themselves? Of course not. Extensive research has been done on the qualities or characteristics that are considered universally attractive. Of them, perhaps the most important is confidence. Confidence, more than anything else, is supremely attractive to women. When we stop taking care of ourselves, our confidence takes a beating. The inevitable outcome is that our partners lose their feelings of attraction to us.

What's more, when you stop taking care of yourself, your wife will begin to see it as a lack of care for her. She may begin to tell herself that you don't love her and that she doesn't matter to you. Needless to say, when our wives begin to feel as though they don't matter to us, they will begin to detach from the relationship. We may not end up dealing with an affair or getting a divorce, but our marriages will begin the downward slide into undesirable places.

BE THE KING OF YOUR CASTLE

Adult romantic love, despite our wishes, is not unconditional. Mature masculine men understand that fully. Adult romantic love is an ongoing, and usually unspoken, negotiation process wherein each person assesses how the relationship feels to them. When we think about loving relationships this way, it casts them in a light that makes them more fragile, more honest, and ultimately more available to greater levels of satisfaction. If adult romantic love was purely unconditional, I wouldn't have had to sit through agonizing counseling sessions with hundreds of men whose wives left them because they weren't being nurtured in the relationship anymore. I'm not giving an unfair view of marriage, but simply a realistic appraisal. I've seen too many husbands give up on taking care of themselves shortly after becoming married – only to be surprised when the marriage is in the gutter. The mature masculine man cherishes the marriage relationship and cherishes himself enough to be mindful of putting his best foot forward. He's not resting in an immature hope that his partner will adore him, admire him, and want to have sex with him, even though he isn't acting in a way that's adorable, admirable, or sexually appealing.

The mature masculine man carries himself through society in such a way that honors himself and honors his wife. Black Belt Husbands are the kings of their castle, and assume this role with great pride. Black Belt Husbands see their wives as cherished additions to their lives and they'll never let another man become the object of their wife's attention. As the cliché goes, "if you never want your wife to leave you, be the kind of husband that is un-leavable". Being that kind of husband means carrying ourselves with pride, self-respect, and dignity in all that we do. We do it because we see the much deeper meaning, as opposed to believing it's simply about appearance.

A BLACK BELT HUSBAND SAYS NO TO DAD BOD

How are you doing in this area, guys? Are you the king of your castle, walking tall with a sense of dignity and pride? The kind of king that wears his golden crown adorned with jewels? The kind of king that is deserving of respect, because he has so much self-respect? Or, if you're honest with yourself, are you a sloppy king? Go through the questions below and give yourself an honest assessment. They may provoke a defensive reaction when you read them because they can feel shaming. Remember, we're not here to judge ourselves harshly. We simply want to make an honest appraisal of where we're at on the journey to Black Belt Husband.

- Has your wife ever accused you of being too fat, or not looking your best? These comments can sting. When you see them as your wife's attempt to communicate that she feels unimportant to you, they become less personal and usually sting less. Have you made this connection with her complaints and feelings about the marriage?
- In your most objective self-analysis, do you try as hard to impress your wife today as you did when you were first together? If the answer is no, why do you think you stopped? Do you think your pulling back has contributed to the current state of your marriage?
- Do you carry yourself in a way that impresses your wife or makes her proud? Or conversely, is she embarrassed by you at times?

- Knowing that self-confidence is the bedrock of human attractiveness, do you carry yourself as someone with lots of self-confidence?
- It's important that we're impressed by our partners in adult romantic relationships. Are you impressive to your wife? Does she brag about you?
- The term "dad bod" has received a lot of publicity lately. It's a term to describe how men put on weight as they become new dads. It's a playful, but disparaging word and not a title we want to carry, despite its seeming innocence. Do you fit in the dad bod category?
- A lot of guys struggle with feeling that their wives don't respect them. In your own analysis of yourself, do you think you live your life and carry yourself in a way that is worthy of respect?
- It's important to remember that we're not talking about vanity; what we want is to impress our wives with our own self-respect, which translates to some powerful emotions for her. With that in mind, when was the last time you did a wardrobe overhaul and updated your sense of fashion? Again, it's not about the vanity.
- Your wife interprets your self-care as a reflection of your care for her. How can you take better care of yourself which in turn will communicate to her that she really matters to you?

These questions, when read at face value, might seem superficial, but I assure you they aren't. In a world that has become hyper-sensitive about not saying the wrong thing, people often feel like these topics are off-limits. Yet, every time we label conversations about physical appearance being off-limits, we suppress an honest engagement about real feelings. Your wife may not feel comfortable talking about these things with you, but that doesn't mean she feels great about everything. You have to make an honest appraisal of yourself.

BLACK BELT HUSBAND TRAINING: MAKING HER FEEL LIKE A QUEEN

Black Belt Husbands are not paranoid or anxious about their appearance, but they are mindful of the implications and so carry themselves with pride. They're not continually obsessing over every little thing. And instead of living with a ton of anxiety that you have to get it perfect, I simply want you to adopt the mentality of a king. Like any good king, you want to impress your queen. So what kinds of things can you do to portray the image of kingship in your marriage? The twenty-first century king is full of self-respect, and his self-respect garners the respect of others. The twenty-first century king sees his queen as worthy of his honor. His pride for himself and for her is shown in very simple ways. These are important elements on the path to Black Belt Husband.

You might read this list and be tempted to dismiss its significance. You might want to chalk it up to superficial vanity. Don't do that! These things carry a lot of weight in your marriage and are deeply meaningful.

Pride in Grooming

Instead of wearing that grimy, sweat stained baseball hat, make an appointment to get your hair cut. Or better yet, make a standing appointment to get your hair cut every other week or once every month. A stylish haircut will go a long way with your queen if it's something you haven't done in a while. When was the last time you spent money on a good cologne or cared about how you smell? If it's been a while, it's worth revisiting. There is very interesting research that suggests the sense of smell is closely linked to libido. It may be time to consider if your scent is bringing her closer to you or pushing her away.

Pride in Physique

When was the last time you really made a concerted effort to get back in shape? Or when was the last time you consistently participated in a physically strenuous activity? Your physique matters, and if you're overweight, it matters to your wife. You don't need to be a male fitness model but being obese is not Black Belt Husband material. I know that might sound harsh, but I have to be honest. Women love fit men who take good care of their bodies. They like an attractive physique when they are dating you in the beginning and they like an attractive physique twenty years later. Women are sexual beings and are attracted, just like men, to quality physical appearance. Can you consider hiring a personal trainer and a nutritionist to help you get back in control of your physique? That's what Black Belt Husbands do because they know it matters.

Pride in Style

Before you accuse me of trying to make you metrosexual, just know I'm not. You don't have to shop at Banana Republic, but you have to care about what you wear. Could you imagine the President of the United States wearing a suit that looked like it came from the Salvation Army? Of course not. Or could you imagine a CEO of a Fortune 500 company wearing shoes that were torn and tattered? Of course not. You are the President and CEO of your home and it's important to dress like it. Your queen is being devalued by anything less.

At first pass, this list may read as trivial, superficial nonsense. You may even be irritated that I wrote it. I understand that it can come across as judgmental and shaming. That's not my intention, but I do feel the need to tell you some hard things and why these things matter. You might even be thinking, "these things can't be that important". Remember, carrying yourself as a king sends a loud and powerful message to your queen. You're either communicating that she is prized and worthy of great respect or you're communicating that she's not worth impressing.

Moving from ultra-intentional habits when you first dated to laziness and neglect is one of the most common, easy and overlooked reasons why woman begin detaching in marriage.

What may seem like trivial things to you - staying fit, being properly groomed, etc. - actually communicate quite a bit and evoke feelings in your queen that are deeply powerful. It's not trivial at all.

MORE SELF RESPECT LEADS TO MORE OF HER RESPECT

As you embrace your role as king, and begin living like a king, some really cool things will happen in your marriage. For starters, and most importantly, you'll begin to feel better about yourself when you take better care of yourself. You'll have more self-confidence. When your confidence increases, you become more secure in just about every area of your life. Your work life improves. Your relationship with your children deepens. You interact with your spouse from a place of strength and dignity, which fosters a greater degree of her earned respect. I've worked with many men over the years who desperately yearn for the respect of their wives.

But respect is earned, not simply given. And just like black belts in BJJ who spend a lifetime perfecting being assassins and earning the respect of others, so it is with Black Belt Husbands.

Many men don't operate as kings, but want to be respected like kings. It's impossible for any of us, including our wives, to fake a feeling of respect when it isn't there. When you start acting like a king and operating from a place of nobility, it brings forward the respect of others, especially your wife. She will begin to admire and respect you. Who wouldn't want more of that?

When you start acting like a king - with pride, dignity, and self-respect - your wife interprets these actions as one of the ways you show you care for her. Even a simple act like being well groomed carries an implicit message that says, "You are important to me". Conversely, if you are not well groomed, the risk is that the implicit message goes something like, "He doesn't care about me". When looking at this simple act through a lens of risk and reward, the risk doesn't seem to make good sense. If something as simple as being well groomed shows your queen that you love her, then do more of it. Your wife wants to feel like she is the apple of your eye.

When you take good care of yourself, you communicate to her that she matters to you. As you get better at living like a king, your wife will begin to feel more secure in the relationship. When she feels more secure, she's going to be able to reciprocate your love. If you want her to act like a queen, you need to first act like a king.

BLUE BELT SKILLS TEST

PRACTICAL SKILL NEEDED TO MOVE FORWARD

Becoming a Black Belt Husband is sometimes about learning new things and sometimes about remembering old things. When you first met your wife, you dated her. Passionately. You went out of your way to impress her. If you're like many guys, you eventually got complacent, and this is a cancer eating away at the relationship. In order to become a Black Belt Husband, you can't be complacent. It's not good for you, it's not good for your wife, and it's not good for your relationship. In order to change the tide, you have to re-learn how to date your wife.

Required Skill: Date Your Wife For Thirty Days

Over the next thirty days, I want you to go into a metaphorical time capsule and do all the things you did when you were first dating your wife. That probably means that you're going to try and look your best. You're going to be well groomed and you're going to be appropriately self-conscious. You're going to clean your car. You're going to get a new outfit for your date with her. You're going to be on time. You're going to hit the gym to lose those extra pounds. You're going to get new underwear and socks. Your marriage deserves this simple effort from you. These are easy, underhand pitches. If you do this over a thirty-day period, your wife is going to notice. I promise. She's going to appreciate your effort immensely. Even if she doesn't say anything, she's watching. If you do this for thirty days, my promise is that it's going to shift the energy in your marriage for the better.

BLUE BELT ATTRIBUTES SUMMARY

Before we move on to purple belt, let's recap a summary of what we've learned in blue belt. Blue belt is all about gaining internal strength and learning to reclaim our birthright of self-confidence. Growing in self-confidence comes from a commitment to honesty, assertiveness, and pride in the way we carry ourselves. The blue belt journey is about challenging our comfort and complacency for the betterment of ourselves and our marriages. During the blue belt journey, we might get a few bumps and bruises along the way, but it's a necessary part of laying the foundation for a marriage that's unstoppable.

Blue Belt I—Honesty Summary:

Before we can attempt to be leaders in our marriage (the stuff of later chapters), we have to first be honest about what is important to us. Self-denial from a fear of conflict is what leads to resentment and all sorts of other problems in marriage. We must be honest about who we are, what is important to us, and what we want out of life and marriage. These conversations may lead to conflict, but without them we're resigning ourselves to a dissatisfying marriage. Marital discontent is inevitable if we're dishonest because we fear conflict.

Blue Belt II—Assertiveness Summary:

Honesty in marriage is about recognizing what is important to us and speaking up about it. The next step, assertiveness, is about taking our honesty and putting it into action by holding ourselves responsible for our own needs. Lovingly insisting that we prioritize ourselves by killing the horrendous people pleaser that will drain our souls. Being more assertive means taking ownership of our lives and recognizing that we are ultimately responsible for the happiness we experience in our marriage.

Blue Belt III—Pride Summary:

When we're more honest, assertive, and putting in the work we learned from section one, we begin to feel more pride in ourselves and what matters to us. We can carry ourselves with strength and dignity. We're reminded in this section that Black Belt Husbands are the kings of their castles and carry themselves as such. Carrying ourselves with pride goes well below the surface as a deeply meaningful gesture and communicates to our wives they are valued and treasured.

Congratulations!
You've graduated from Blue Belt!

SECTION THREE

The Purple Belt Journey; Becoming Well-Rounded In Our Craft

For to win one hundred victories in one hundred battles is not the acme of skill. To subdue the enemy without fighting is the acme of skill.

—Sun Tzu, *The Art of War*

WELCOME TO PURPLE BELT

The purple belt journey is about refining our skillsets as husbands in ways that separate us from the pack of everyday husbands. In our blue belt work, we focused on being true to ourselves, which grows our strength and self-confidence. Now and only now can we build upon that strength to offer our partners an experience that turns our relationship into something sought after and envied by the masses. The purple belt journey is exciting because we begin to experience our relationship as flowing and tension-free, often for the first time.

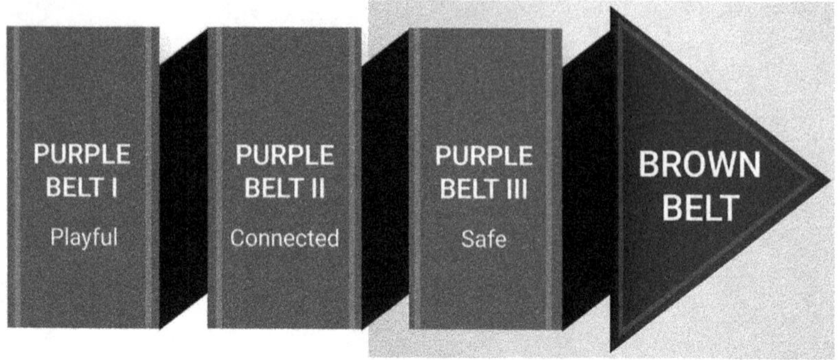

CHAPTER 7

Purple Belt I: Playful; Being the Safe Harbor in Her Storm

PLAY IS THE ANTIDOTE TO STRESS

By the time you have reached purple belt in BJJ - usually after five years of dedicated training - you have enough self-confidence in your abilities as a grappler that you're able to begin taking more subtle risks in your jiu-jitsu game. Purple belts in jiu-jitsu have enough fundamentals down that they can become more playful. Purple belts on the journey to Black Belt Husbands mirror the jiu-jitsu path in that they also become more playful as husbands. Jiu-jitsu purple belts have less to prove to others because they're grounded in their own self-confidence. Similarly, the purple belt journey en route to Black Belt Husband opens the door for more play, spontaneity, and lightheartedness in marriage. The purple belt is rooted in skills that come from lower ranking belts—honesty, self-awareness, assertiveness, humility, etc. As a result, he can open himself to being more playful in marriage.

For the average husband, it can be hard to find a sense of playfulness. It's not uncommon for many husbands to be filled with mountains of stress, worry, and anxieties that are eroding to their marriage. Even subtle, ambient levels of worry—most often related to work stress—create a kind of tension and rigidity that can bleed into relationships. Things can just feel tense and uneasy. For many men, the concept of being playful and having spontaneous fun has escaped them for so long that they may not even realize it's missing. Certainly, many men feel lost about how to course correct and add more playfulness into their lives.

When I was studying clinical psychology in graduate school, I remember sitting through a child development class and learning how to assess for psychological problems in children. Children, when suffering from too much stress, will be most impacted in their inability to spontaneously play, and child psychologists observe playfulness (or lack of) as a way of assessing the severity of psychological problems.

When children have a hard time playing, it's a sign that something is wrong. The same concepts about children's play can also be applied to adults. Although not commonly discussed, the psychological health of adults can be assessed by observing their ability or inability to spontaneously play. Adults, like children, cannot live playfully, spontaneously, or lightheartedly, when they are suffering from a mountain of stress. Stress, worry, and anxiety undermine the possibility of authentic play for men. So we become uptight, rigid, and angry in turn. Snapping at our kids for innocent mistakes.

An excess of stress and a lack of play will affect every relationship over time. Things may feel tense, too serious, and void of the necessary joy that relationships should bring. Since many men disproportionately see their role in marriage as that of financial providers, their stress about work can become all-consuming and interfere with opportunities to be playful and just connect. In order to compensate for day-to-day stress and tension, many men will book an exotic vacation a few times a year. Still, it's never enough to make up for the thousand lost opportunities for play daily and spontaneously. What's more, stress is often the root cause of alcoholism or other forms of substance abuse. But as you know, those cocktails may temporarily alleviate the stress, but the relief never lasts. Absent these moments of temporary relief, however, many men would feel completely shackled by the seriousness of their lives. Black Belt Husbands experience stress too, just like anyone else. Yet they know how to turn it on and turn it off and they know when they're reaching their tipping point and when they're at capacity. Black Belt Husbands know when to buckle down and solve serious problems, but they're mindful that the seriousness of life doesn't cripple their relationships along the way. Black Belt Husbands see the need for spontaneous play in their lives and in their marriages.

BEING PLAYFUL MAKES US MAGNETIZING HUSBANDS

Have you ever spent time around someone that took themselves too seriously? They don't feel good to be around. I'm guilty of it. My work as a therapist requires that I spend much of my waking hours being entrenched in the challenges that others are experiencing. There is a level of seriousness in my work that bleeds into my life at home and my relationship with my friends and family if I do not commit to turning it off. My mind can easily get lost and distracted thinking about my clients and how best to help them. So much so that I can forget to smile and just enjoy the goodness of life with a sense of ease. To be honest, being playful actually takes a lot of effort for me. And I know my work stress isn't unique either. Most of my clients have high-stress and demanding jobs that can easily kill their joy too.

For the sake of your marriage, you need to wonder about, and guard against, any tendency to show up in your relationship too serious. The benefit of marriage, beyond the satisfaction of basic physical and safety needs, is to offer two people a partnership in which they can experience an improved quality of life together. Part of the improved quality of life is the experience of being joyful and playful with each other. When you are consumed with too much stress, the natural outcome is that you simply aren't fun to be around. Of course, being uptight and rigid is not your true essence. You know how to be light hearted and have fun. But you may have forgotten how important it is. Or, you might have a hard time giving yourself permission to do so. If life has become too stressful for you and too filled with worries, it's time to reevaluate because your relationship isn't sustainable like this.

In this chapter, we are reminding ourselves to value the fact that our wives want to have fun with us. They want to see us smile, naturally and spontaneously. And they want us to be a beacon of light during dark days. Your wife wants to play with you. She wants to laugh with you and be joyful alongside you. I know you want that too. We all do.

When you're able to become more spontaneously playful, you offer your wife an experience that she craves. As you learn to be more playful, you become a refuge for your wife in her challenging times. Black Belt Husbands have the ability to be spontaneously playful and see the value it provides to their marriage. They have a confidence that allows them to lower their guard, set aside, or deal with the anxieties that cause them to not show up in the marriage in the best way possible.

WITHOUT SPONTANEOUS PLAY, WE MISS PRECIOUS MOMENTS TO CONNECT

For men who struggle with being playful, it's commonly a result of the strain of life causing them to lose their childlike spirit somewhere along the road. We want to keep our childlike spirit, which differs from immaturity or childish behavior. The childlike spark I'm describing keeps us curious, spontaneous, playful, and joyful in life. These are the most beautiful attributes we all admire. The reason children can do it so well, usually much more naturally than adults, is because they are totally in the moment. They aren't thinking about yesterday or tomorrow. They aren't obsessing about that project they need to finish at work. Children are masters of being present.

When we forego being present, we negatively impact our marriages. If we're stressed, worried, or obsessing about this other thing or that other thing, we miss the precious moments in life. No matter how hard we try, we simply can't have fun if our minds are consumed with anxious thoughts. We may try to fake it, but it never works. Our wives want to have fun with us. They want to be light-hearted, make jokes, laugh, and play with us. That's part of why they married us. And we want to share these same experiences with them. When life becomes so intense that we miss these moments, we're neglecting an important aspect of successful relationships.

I've worked with many couples that have struggled with infidelity. The lack of play in these relationships has been a common denominator in almost every case. When playfulness disappears from a relationship for too long, there is always a yearning to find it again, somewhere, even if outside the relationship. We look for fun, light-heartedness, and spontaneity. When I ask the cheating partner how an affair started, it always begins the same way. Someone other than the spouse is playful with them. It starts as a playful smile, a light hello, and progresses to a shared laugh, etc. Over time, two people, not even with bad intentions are sincerely enjoying each other with lightness, laughter, and the kind of joy that makes us feel alive. Playfulness is often synonymous with chemistry that people refer to when they talk about being attracted to one another. And when it's missing from a relationship for too long, we risk that our partners may experience it with someone else.

The parents of one of my closest friends were celebrating their sixtieth wedding anniversary and they invited me to their party. I was honored to celebrate such a milestone because you don't get to see something so significant every day and I couldn't wait to go. The party was on a Saturday night and when I arrived I quickly noticed that hundreds of cars lined the streets outside the house. After driving around for thirty minutes looking for a place to park, I realized this wasn't going to be the quaint, quiet, intimate gathering I had imagined. My friends happen to be Puerto Rican, and if you've ever been lucky enough to hang with people from this island, you know that they know how to have a great time. There were crowds of people, loud music, food, drinking, and lots of salsa dancing. It was an incredible party that would have rivaled any party I attended in my twenties.

What was interesting about this party was that it was a celebration of two people in their mid-eighties celebrating sixty years of marriage. And they were at the center of the celebration - leading the charge. They weren't on the periphery of the party - they were front and center. It wasn't a party for them, they were running it! They were pulling people half their age onto the dance floor. They were taking shots with their grandchildren. They were running around opening beers and making cocktails for the "young people" in their fifties.

The party went all night in full force and a little after midnight I could see the couple getting ready to leave. As the party was winding down, I mentioned to my friend, their son, that it was fun to be at the event and remarked about how tired his parents must be. My friend looked at me and said, "Are you kidding? They are driving to the casino now to go gamble". I was stunned! A couple in their eighties, married for sixty years, partying all night and heading off to the casino to gamble after midnight. The event that night was etched into my memory because I didn't know that being so playful was a possibility after a marriage of sixty years. My parents certainly didn't model that type of playfulness and I was truly captivated by it. This couple held onto the magic of play that so many of us seem to lose. For sixty years of marriage, this couple continued to enjoy each other, life, and their love for spontaneous play. When was the last time you played that way?

NEVER GIVE A SWORD TO A MAN WHO CAN'T DANCE

Playfulness is a state of mind that says, "I'm willing to shut out everything else and enjoy the moment". Free of anxiety and worry, we open ourselves up to being truly present with our partners for moments of joy. The mature masculine man is what I call a multidimensional man. He has the ability to be fierce when called upon and the ability to be playful when called upon. Multidimensional men understand that the masculine journey is much more robust than simply being a stoic, serious-about-life, income earner. To live in this one-dimensional place yields very little life satisfaction for yourself or your family apart from accumulated material possessions that we all know mean very little in the end. The mature masculine understands that stress, worry, and anxiety are simply part of life and sees the need for working with them in a way that doesn't rob him of his capacity for play.

The mature masculine man, in his fullest expression is wild and playful. Unlike the stereotypical subdued husband we encounter most often and are at risk of becoming. The mature masculine man is untamed. He isn't worried about offending others with his spontaneity and he doesn't obsess about looking so put together that he forgets to enjoy the moment. The mature masculine lives life in full color. He is playful, spontaneous, fun, and does not take himself too seriously. He knows how to offer his family the joy they need from him. The mature masculine man embodies the Celtic proverb that reads: "Never give a sword to a man that can't dance" which references our playful dimension preceding our warrior dimension.

HOW SERIOUS HAS LIFE BECOME FOR YOU?

Many men are buried under the pressures of life and eventually lose their capacity for playfulness. Stress and worry have created a lack of vitality. When life becomes an event to numb from, we can be sure we've been robbed of our wild and playful spirit. No work stress, mortgage payment, or potential promotion is worth sacrificing our ability to enjoy life and the people important to us. Take a look at some of the questions below and assess your own level of spontaneity, being present, and playfulness.

- When you look at the amount of time we spend thinking about your work and time spent at work, does it feel disproportionately out of balance with the amount of time you spend enjoying your life?
- On average between Monday and Friday, how often would your wife say that you are enjoyable to be around?
- Are you struggling with stress, worry, and anxiety? How long has it been this way? Do you think this is sustainable to live this way?
- Do you find yourself drinking alcohol as a way of escaping from the stressors of everyday life? Does drinking offer you that temporary moment of happiness that you might not feel otherwise?
- I know there can be a temptation to blame others (primarily your wife) for your discontent, but only you are responsible for your own happiness. What do you do on a consistent basis to make yourself happy?
- If you're a dad and you're really honest with yourself, are your children going to remember how playful you were or how distracted you seemed?
- When I use the term wild, I'm referring to that part of us that is not totally put together in a perfectionistic

way. Being playful requires us to tap into our wild side with a bit of reckless abandon. When was the last time you did something really wild?

- In your honest assessment, how much energy do you put into image management and showcasing to the world that you have it all together? Knowing this facade of perfectionism is the death knell of playfulness, what stands in the way of your beginning to shed it?

BLACK BELT HUSBAND TRAINING: WHO WERE YOU AS A KID? WHERE DID *HE* GO?

When I was young I used to love going on long bike rides with my neighborhood friends. In practicality, we wouldn't go very far - maybe only a few blocks or so - but to us it felt like we'd ventured miles away. On these bike rides, we were living in the moment. We were adventurous. We were wild and playful. I loved that time from my childhood and some of my fondest memories as a kid were these adventures with my friends. But during adulthood, I lost my sense of playfulness. Life got too intense and serious for me and I was weighed down by the pressure to succeed. I drove a nice car and wore nice suits, but I wasn't playing anymore. When I woke to the reality that I was discontent with the life I had created for myself, I began reflecting on my experiences as a kid and what I used to love doing. Feeling burdened by the stresses of day-to-day life, I longed for those days of spontaneity and freedom. I daydreamed, with envy, about the adventurous bike rides with my friends. I was motivated to begin playing again and I looked to my past to help me reclaim my playfulness. Looking in the rearview mirror of our lives can become the path to reclaim our sense of play.

What did you love to do as a kid? What kinds of games did you love playing? What adventures did you love to go on? The answers to these questions are the keys to unlocking your own suppressed playfulness. When we were kids, we had no problem playing. We didn't know any other way to live life. We had no worries and we didn't need to pretend to have it all together. Then, of course, life happens and we begin believing the lie that playing is the stuff of children. Then we become sick with anxiety and depression and wonder why we're not happy and our wives don't want to spend time with us. To free ourselves of the rigidity, boredom, and stagnation of adult life, we need to go back in time and remember what we used to love doing. How can we begin recreating those loves in our lives today? To see how it works, and for the purpose of reference, here are a few examples of connecting my childhood to my adulthood in the realm of play:

- As a kid, I loved playing with guns and participating in games of cops and robbers. As an adult, I'm an avid shooter and modest gun collector. Shooting with my friends is just as exhilarating and exciting as I remember it when I was young.
- As a kid, I loved to wrestle with my brother, my sister, and my friends. As an adult, I love training in Brazilian jiu-jitsu. It reminds me of being a kid again and brings the same amount of joy.
- As a kid, I loved those long bike rides in the neighborhood. As an adult, I love trail riding on my dirt bike. My riding friends and I will go for days and get lost in the wilderness on our motorcycles. This is the adult version of those magical neighborhood bike rides when I was a kid.

These are just a few personal examples of how my childhood loves play out in my own life. I could go on and tell you how it also relates to playing golf, surfing, mountain biking, trail running, my love for photography, or restoring furniture. Are you able to see the connection? So, what is it for you? What did you love doing when you were young? And how can you reclaim that in your life today? I can tell you with great conviction that when I interact with my wife and family after playing, I am present, usually dirty, and so content that it directly and positively impacts my marriage. My wife is the beneficiary of my play too.

PLAYFULNESS IS AN ASSET AND TOO MUCH SERIOUSNESS BECOMES A LIABILITY

When we reduce our stress, worry, and anxiety, we are enjoyable to be around. It's really that simple. When you're playful, you feel relaxed, calm, and present; you become an asset to your wife's life. Of course, you need to give yourself permission to have bad days. But what I'm talking about in this chapter is something more pervasive and constant that can go missing in our lives for too long.

Life can be very tough sometimes. We go out in the world and sometimes feel beat up. We want to be able to see our partners as the safe harbor in the storm of life. A place that can reduce our stress. When we're so tense and serious we're no longer that safe harbor in the storm.

Being playful isn't about making bad jokes or refusing to have serious and important conversations when they're necessary. Being playful is a state of mind that brings a smile to your wife's face because she knows you will be an emotional asset to her when she needs you to be playful.

PURPLE BELT SKILLS TEST

PRACTICAL SKILL NEEDED TO MOVE FORWARD

If we're to become more playful, we need to address the stress, worry and perfectionism that get in the way. And one of the best ways to tackle this type of unhelpful thinking is with mindfulness practices. Although mindfulness sounds like a fancy word, it's actually really simple. It's a type of self-talk that can help ground us in the present moment by reminding us of what is true. Too often, the worries we obsess about are not grounded in reality, but in negative thoughts that are inaccurate and keep us on edge. Mindfulness practices will break this bad habit.

Required Skill: Thirty Days of Mindfulness Before You Arrive Home

Over the next thirty days, I want you to find just five minutes to read this script before you come home from work for the day. Find a quiet place, even if it's sitting in your car, take several relaxed breathes, and read this script to yourself calmly and slowly. When you do so repeatedly over the course of a month, you'll notice how much calm and relaxation you feel. As you begin to feel more calm and relaxed, playfulness is the natural byproduct.

I'm Okay (a mindfulness script to reduce stress)

{Your name}, you move at a very fast pace
You need to slow down if you want to connect with {Her name}
You expect a lot out of people, sometimes too much
This keeps you isolated and disconnected
{Your name}, you are strong and brave.
{Your name}, you are okay
You are more than okay, you are doing really well.
You can relax and enjoy the goodness of this present moment.

{Your name}, You are solid
You are as solid as a mountain
And you can rest knowing you are very loved and cared for
{Your name}, you are okay
{Your name}, you can be playful like you were when you were a child
That child still lives inside you and wants to play again.
He is safe enough to come out and play
{Your name}, the little boy inside you is going to be okay.
Nobody will die
You are not in harm's way
Whatever it is you worry about will work itself out.
It will all be okay
Urgency is not helpful right now
More patience is what you need
Your wife wants to smile with you.
You can smile with her.
{Your name} You will be okay.

CHAPTER 8

Purple Belt II: Connected; Building a Band of Brothers Who Stand Together

WE CAN'T DO IT ALONE

Becoming a Black Belt Husband requires us to be connected to a band of brothers made up of other like-minded husbands. Black Belt Husbands know they can't do the marriage journey alone and need the connectivity of other men to keep them on the right path.

Too often, the modern married man is supremely isolated from authentic male friendship and genuine accountability. Being connected with other like-minded men offers us benefits such as support, confidence, accountability, and relatability. Yet, despite the enormous benefit and critical importance of genuine male friendships, so few men actually have them. When we lack an inner circle of male friendship, we're left to figure things out for ourselves. Needless to say, this rarely ends positively.

After interviewing all the men I've worked with in my practice over the years, I've learned that only about 20 percent of them have what I would call an inner circle of male friends in whom they can confide about life's most difficult challenges. That means eight out of ten guys are trying to do it on their own; unsuccessfully stumbling in the dark. The majority of men, when asked about their male friendships, will speak of buddies they see when watching sporting events, talking about business, or playing golf. That's usually where the relationship seems to end. Very few men have male friends with whom they can share their life struggles and that's a huge problem as it keeps the modern man extremely isolated from other men. Throughout the history of time, men have always banded together and shared burdens of life. But in our modern civilization, the idea of men connecting with each other through life's challenges is looked upon as something that is weak or unmanly. In pop culture, we jokingly poke fun at male friendship and call it "bromance". Somehow, sadly, two men being open and honest with each other is jokingly analogous to a homosexual relationship.

Despite our heroic attempts to have it all together and not need anyone's help, we are in desperate need of a band of brothers to share the burdens of life with us. Any man who tells you he can do it on his own without the support of others is either hiding behind his facade of perfectionism or entrenched in his own delusion. By the time we get to purple belt on our way toward Black Belt Husband, we have to see the need for authentic male friendship to carry us through the rest of the way on the journey. We can't do it alone, no matter how great we believe in our self-reliance. Living in isolation from an inner circle is white belt stuff. Successfully navigating purple belt work requires that we change this aspect of our lives. Being a successful husband is not an individual effort. It's a community affair and we need to be able to rely on one another if we're going to pull it off.

In fact, Black Belt Husbands are supremely connected to other men. They have a tribe of men they can call and rely upon. They do so not only to share in the successes of life, but also to open up about life's challenges. Black Belt Husbands value authentic relationships with other like-minded men who share similar values in life, relationships, and marriage. Black Belt Husbands approach life with an understanding that they need to be accountable to, and challenged by their inner circle. Otherwise, they know that they are at risk to move through life making choices and acting in ways that are out of alignment with their own core values. No matter how resolute and steadfast we believe ourselves to be, all of us face the risk of veering from the path. Sometimes, even the best of us need someone to tell us we're way off course. We need our tribe to keep us moving in the right direction.

BEING SUCCESSFUL IN MARRIAGE REQUIRES US TO BE CONNECTED TO A BAND OF BROTHERS

If we lack having our own inner circle of authentic male friends, where do we turn for reality-testing to assess what is happening in our marriage? How do we know if what's happening for us is good or bad, sane or insane, healthy or unhealthy? Without the connectedness of a community of brothers, we're left to ourselves to make sense of things, which can very often end badly.

All of us have our own blind spots, places where we don't see ourselves accurately. We need a band of brothers to help us see more clearly. Unfortunately, we live in a culture that promotes individualism over community and self-sufficiency over interdependence, especially for men. Men are told that relying emotionally on other men is a sign of weakness. And this is killing men and marriages.

What a tragic lie, however. Because the truth is that it takes a significantly stronger man to rely on the input from another man than it does for any man to pretend he can do it alone. Married men need good friends and need them badly. Good friends, life-giving friends that can help them feel connected to one another when things get turbulent in life and in marriage.

We have to challenge the conventional wisdom that promotes the idea that we can and must handle it on our own as "strong men".

There are innumerable benefits to having a band of brothers. Without enumerating them all in an exhaustive list, here is a brief overview of five of the most important elements that the inner circle offers us.

A Place to Confide In

There is something very powerful about being able to confide in another man about our innermost thoughts and perceptions. There is a saying in the field of clinical psychology, "we're only as sick as our secrets". If we don't have the type of male friendships where we can confide in someone else, we risk holding things inside through an emotionally destructive suppression process. When we do this, we're creating a mountain of future psychological problems.

A Place to Feel Relatable

It's a basic human tendency to believe that we're the only ones who are experiencing certain hardships in life. When things are not going well, it's common for people to think, "I don't think anyone else is going through this but me". It's hard to imagine that other married men experience similar hardships, but they do. I do. We all do. When we come to realize we're not the only ones fighting the fight, it feels like a thousand-pound weight lifted off our shoulders.

A Place for Emotional Diversity

Many married men have a tendency to lean too heavily on their spouses for support, encouragement, and reassurance. There can be a risk of putting too many emotional eggs in our spouse's basket. Men, your wife cannot be your everything despite pop culture's hideous insistence that marriage is supposed to serve all our needs. At the same time, we can't do it all by ourselves either, which is the other end of the spectrum for many men. This only leaves us with one option: Emotionally relying on other male friends. When we rely too heavily on our spouses to be the catch all of our emotional life, we are setting ourselves up for disappointment from an impossible expectation. When we're not connected to our inner circle of males, we put a disproportionate amount of expectations on our partners. Developing your inner circle will take the pressure off relying too heavily on your spouse.

A Place for Guidance

Married men need the band of brothers to show them the way through the storms of life. Sometimes, we need to be pointed in the right direction. Black Belt Husbands rely on their tribe as mentors and advisors – the ones that they trust and turn to for practical advice and suggestions. We need these types of authentic friendships to keep ourselves on a healthy path because we all have a tendency to veer from time to time. We can't go through life on our own without a band of brothers showing us the way. The band of brothers are fellow travelers.

A Place to Feel Normal

And lastly, men need the band of brothers to normalize the occasional craziness of married life. Being on the marriage journey can bring up all sorts of doubts, confusions, twists and turns. We need good friends along the way to help us realize that what is happening to us is normal. Without the band of brothers normalizing our experiences, we're likely to hit the panic button during times when we'd be better served by taking a deep breath and talking it through with someone we trust.

The importance of being connected to a tribe of other like-minded men can't be overstated. Yet so few men have these types of relationships. Although there is a temptation in saying, "I'm too busy for this", we have to see the potential peril that can arise when we don't have it. Most men have friends with whom they can share hobbies and interests with. And of course, there's nothing wrong with these friendships; they can be really great. Still, we need more. Black Belt Husbands see the critical necessity to move beyond the limited benefit of these types of friendships. Having a band of brothers is something that every man desires deep within, though only a few are brave enough to take the risks necessary to obtain it.

WITHOUT A BAND OF BROTHERS, WE'RE LEFT TO FIGURE THINGS OUT ON OUR OWN

When we lack the important inner circle of male friendship, we miss out on one of the most important and life-giving aspects of being human. Male friendship, rooted in authenticity and honesty, is a gift and an experience that makes life worth living. Without our inner circle, life becomes flat, stale, and mundane. When we look to our experiences as kids to formulate what matters to us also as adults, we can easily see that the most treasured times during our youth were when we banded together with our childhood playmates. Being with our friends when we were young made us feel alive. But many of us grow up and we're told that we need to be responsible, pay the bills, and buckle down into the seriousness of life. With this mindset, it's no surprise that many are isolated, anxious, and depressed as a collective group.

I once worked with a client who was on the fence in his marriage. When talking about male friendship, he looked at me with the most sincere and genuine look at asked, "Quentin, do guys my age have friends?" He genuinely didn't know if it was okay for him to have friends.

Real friends.

The question was heart-breaking, but the truth is that it's a question many guys ask. It's a question that I asked too. For most of my adult life, my definition of male friendship centered around some shared hobby, interest, or sporting thing. The idea of having a true male friend, someone to whom I could open up with in a sincere and honest way, wasn't something that I experienced until I was in my thirties. My client's question broke my heart because I could feel his pain living such an isolated life – I had lived it once too. To be so isolated and cut off from real male friendship is a very painful place. Yet many men experience life this way.

The question he asked said a lot about what was broken in his life and his marriage too. The band of brothers that we're speaking about in this chapter is not only okay, it is critical to our personal well-being and marital success. We need the band of brothers for reflection, support, confidence, and accountability when we're veering astray to keep us on the right path. How can any of us be successful in marriage without these types of relationships? It's rarely possible. Women often get a bad rap for relying on their husbands to be their everything. But men do it too just in a little different way; without the band of brothers, we'll always be at risk for it. When husbands don't have a deeply connected band of brothers, they passively and often unconsciously look to their wives to be the sole providers of self-worth. They treat their wives like their mommy's. When we rely on our wives this way, we give them too much power and influence over our well-being.

Black Belt Husbands are very connected to their band of brothers. They know they can't do the marriage journey alone and rely heavily on their inner circle for all kinds of things. When we don't have this type of inner circle, friendships with other males tend to revolve around work, hobbies, or drinking buddies. I'm not judging these types of friendships, but it's important to make a distinction between superficial friends with whom we can shoot the shit and a more deeply rooted band of brothers that we can call in the middle of the night when our lives are falling apart. We are far less lonely and isolated when we have these relationships. They bring us genuine happiness and an experience of being alive. In turn, the benefits of these authentic friendships make us more successful in marriage.

THE BAND OF BROTHERS CONCEPT HAS PASSED THE TEST OF TIME

Wherever you're at with this topic, I invite you into the journey of finding your own tribe of men, wherever that may be. My hope here is simply that you see the need for an honest, authentic, and truly connected band of brothers. From a historical perspective, men have always been associated with other men. The survival of the group has always been dependent upon men in a tribe working together for the betterment of the tribe. The extent to which historical tribes were successful in doing so determined the longevity of the group. We may not be hunting game together anymore, but we're still in great need for the community that like-minded groups of men have always offered.

The modern man is chronically isolated from other men. Society has set up men for failure in this regard and we need to fight against it. Interestingly, most men ditch the idea of friendships with other men around the time they get married. It's as if men have permission from society to have friends up until that point. Part of this dilemma is centered around issues we talked about in blue belt work (honesty about what's important to you); having an inner circle of male friends can be a point of contention in marriage and cause conflict. No matter what, we need to push back against it. Mature masculine men do not need a lot of friends, but they have a few key friends they can rely upon when things get difficult. Masculine men see the need for other men to keep them challenged, accountable, and included in the world of men.

HOW CONNECTED ARE YOU WITH A BAND OF BROTHERS?

So how would you assess your own inner circle of male friendship? Does it exist at all? Do you have some semblance of one but feel it needs some tweaking and improvement? Finding your inner circle of male friends is critical to your success in becoming a Black Belt Husband. You simply can't navigate the marriage experience in isolation. You need a band of brothers to share in the journey with you. Take a few minutes and answer some of these questions to see how you stack up with this area of your life.

- Do you have a tribe of male friends that you can lean on for emotional support when things get tough?
- Do you currently have active relationships with other men holding you accountable to be the best version of yourself in all aspects of your life?
- If something in your life was falling apart right now, to whom would you reach out if it wasn't your wife and family?
- What was your father's role-modeling with male friendships? Did he have good friends that he relied on for support, accountability, and transparency?
- Pop culture refers to male friendships as "bromances", which is a confusing title to attach to male friendship because it infers that male friendships are somehow analogous with romantic relationships. Do you carry stigmas about male friendship or being close with other men?
- Do you have male mentors in your life who you trust for guidance on being a husband?

When it comes to developing a band of brothers, we're trying to stretch ourselves outside of the superficial form of male friendship which is what exists for most guys. Most male friendships are centered around common interests, stages of life, or occupational relatedness. Which by itself isn't bad, except they're often void of deeper connections based on authenticity and genuine transparency. The common denominators that bring most male friends together are not bad, but they aren't enough. We need to take male relationships to a new level where we can be more open, honest, and interdependent. We need to learn how to rely on one another. We have to shed the desire to live as lone wolves and return to the pack with like-minded men. Our inner circle is a critical factor of success on the Black Belt Husband journey.

BLACK BELT HUSBAND TRAINING: BUILDING YOUR BAND OF BROTHERS

In order to develop an active band of brothers, we have to put in some work to get there. No one ever becomes part of a band of brothers by osmosis. It only happens with a lot of intentionality. A common misconception about developing a band of brothers is that other men are not interested.

That couldn't be further from the truth.

Most men are craving deeper and more meaningful relationships with other men, but perhaps like you, are reluctant to reach out and initiate. We fear rejection, criticism, or perceived weakness for desiring better friendships with like-minded men. As a result of these fears, men everywhere are stuck in their own isolation. They want more, but fear reaching out.

To begin developing your band of brothers, the first step is accurately categorizing your current friends. You may already have friends who are great candidates for your band of brothers, so it's best to start there. However, the truth is a number of your friends will not make the cut. Only those friends who share similar values with you around marriage and are willing to take your friendship to new places qualify for band of brothers. When analyzing your current friendships, you can break them down into three distinct categories: fun friends, work friends, and inner circle friends. There will be some overlap between the groups, but by and large they will fall into these three categories.

FUN FRIENDS

These are the guys you seek out when you're doing something fun. These are your drinking buddies, the guys you want around when you're needing to let loose and have a few laughs. These friends serve a very important function in your life. Even so, they may not make the cut into your band of brothers if you don't share core values with them around marriage. It's not necessary for your fun friends to share your core values, but it's indispensable for your band of brothers. I'm not asking you to ditch your fun friends at all. You're just gaining clarity on how to categorize them.

WORK FRIENDS

If you spend quite a bit of time at the office, you probably have developed some close relationships with the guys there. You and your work friends share the common denominator of your obnoxious boss or some of the hard-to-explain new policies and procedures that drive you nuts. Work friends are often the ones that will commiserate with you about work issues. They're valuable to your sanity in your work life and you need them for it. However, it's very important to have clear boundaries between your professional life and your personal life. As a result, work friends are kept at a certain distance from your authentic self and therefore often don't make the cut into the band of brothers.

INNER CIRCLE FRIENDS (BAND OF BROTHERS)

Your band of brothers consists of friends with whom you can have fun; they may also have a similar work life. But what's necessary to make the cut for your band of brothers is that the quality of the relationship with these guys surpasses the common denominators of having fun or sharing in work life. What's unique to your inner circle friends is that these guys share your value system about life and about marriage. Your inner circle consists of the guys who are your trusted confidants. They are going to keep you accountable and won't be afraid to hold you to the right path. These are the guys you're honest with about everything, and they're honest with you.

The first step in developing an inner circle is to begin with your current friendships and spend some time analyzing them. Think about all the guys you have spent time with over the past six months and create a list by writing their names on a piece of paper. Give them a "F" next to their name for fun friend, a "W" next to their name for work friend, or an "I" next to their name for potential inner circle friend. Once you have created your list, pick five guys in the inner circle category that you feel would be the best candidates to build your band of brothers. If you have less than five, just start there. We'll talk momentarily about what to do with these five names.

BEING WELL CONNECTED WITH A TRIBE OF MEN RESULTS IN A BETTER MARRIAGE

When we become connected to a band of brothers, our relationships improve. That's not to say that our wives won't be jealous or frustrated about our relationship with our band of brothers, but in the end genuine relationships with other men can only improve the quality of our lives and our marriages. Our band of brothers confront our bad decisions or help us gain clarity on how we're not living up to our masculine potential. This input improves the quality of our lives and the quality of our marriages.

And our marriage is the beneficiary.

The band of brothers gets to know us, all the while holding our best interests in mind. They are there to help us become the man we say we want to be. We need this because, we can't reach our full potential in isolation, no matter how hard we try or how resilient we believe ourselves to be. All of us have our own blind spots and need the help of others to see ourselves clearly.

When we become well connected with our band of brothers and begin to move out of isolation, our experience of life is more full, complete, and enriching. In turn, we experience more positive emotions. When we're living in isolation and suffering from the emotional burden that comes from being disconnected, it's easy to see our wives as the reason we're so dissatisfied. We feel like crap about our own lives but blame our spouses for a disproportionate share of our discontent. However, chances are that if we were better connected with our band of brothers, our complaints would be significantly reduced.

Whenever I'm working with a guy going through relationship struggles, I always inquire about his band of brothers. I'll say, "tell me about your friends and the close men in your life who are helping you with this dilemma". When I ask this question, I usually get a look that says, "Huh .... why would I do that?" We need these types of relationships because we need to be told we're way off base or reminded that we're getting walked over. Whatever the problem may be, we always run the risk of being out of touch with it when we live in isolation. A band of brothers helps us stay on the path of our core values which can only result in an improved marriage.

PURPLE BELT SKILLS TEST

PRACTICAL SKILL NEEDED TO MOVE FORWARD

A band of brothers is awaiting you, but you're going to have to do some work in order to get there. Instead of waiting and hoping that the right guys magically show up in your life, you're going to create your own band of brothers. You're going to take control of your life and empower yourself to go after the things you want. That is a Black Belt Husband mindset.

Required Skill: Being proactive building your Band of Brothers

When you think about developing an inner circle, you may be overwhelmed by the prospect of finding multiple men for your tribe. But you don't have to do it all at once. Instead, you can start small. I want you to think of just one friend you have right now who shares similar values around life and marriage. Once you have this guy in your head, I want you to reach out to him and say the following (feel free to change the language and make it your own. This is just an example of the core message you're trying to get across):

Hey Joe,

I hope you're doing well.

I've been thinking lately about how I could really benefit from having better and more consistent friendships in my life.

I've been thinking about how it would be cool to have my own "band of brothers" to develop more accountability.

I'm looking for guys who share my core values about marriage, life, etc.

I thought you would be a great person to start with and I'm wondering if you might be interested in working together and helping one another?

Let me know what you think, and if you're interested we can talk more about it. If not, no problem, I understand.

Cheers.

Quentin

The message is short, direct, and conveys that you're wanting to take your friendship to new and more meaningful levels. If your friend says he's not interested, don't take it personally. It's likely that he's simply not ready to go deeper yet. Your job is to start with one friend at a time until you have five guys who have said yes. Then you have your inner circle and are one step closer to Black Belt Husband.

CHAPTER 9

Purple Belt III: Safe; Protecting Her by Being Emotionally Available

MEETING OUR PARTNER WHERE THEY'RE AT

As we near the end of the purple belt journey, we should be moving in the direction of becoming a safe and emotionally protective presence for our partner. Being safe in this regard has nothing to do with physical safety; instead it's about emotional safety. Black Belt Husbands are incredibly safe and offer their partners an emotional experience that helps them feel valued, understood, cared for, and respected.

Several hundred years ago, it was the role and duty of the husband to protect his wife and family from physical threats. There may have been wild animals, competitive tribes, financial ruin, etc. that required the man of the house to offer his physical protection. Safety meant something different in the past than it does today. Today, we may face some of those threats, but for most couples in the twenty-first century, the need to protect against basic physical needs has been greatly diminished. Our role as husbands has graduated from satiating basic physical needs to providing for basic emotional needs.

Instead of helping our partners feel safe from a threat that could jeopardize their basic physical safety, our wives are looking to us to create a sense of safety with them that satisfies deeper, emotional needs. The idea of being a safe emotional presence for our partner can feel perplexing to a lot of guys because for most of us, we haven't been taught how to do this. But when we understand it better, it will begin to make perfect sense. The famous psychologist Abraham Maslow is mostly remembered for his work on the different stages of the human experience which he conceptualized with his hierarchy of needs. He described the human experience as a dynamic journey that moves from fulfilling our most basic and primitive needs like having enough food, water, and shelter, to more complicated needs. Here is a depiction of the hierarchy of needs:

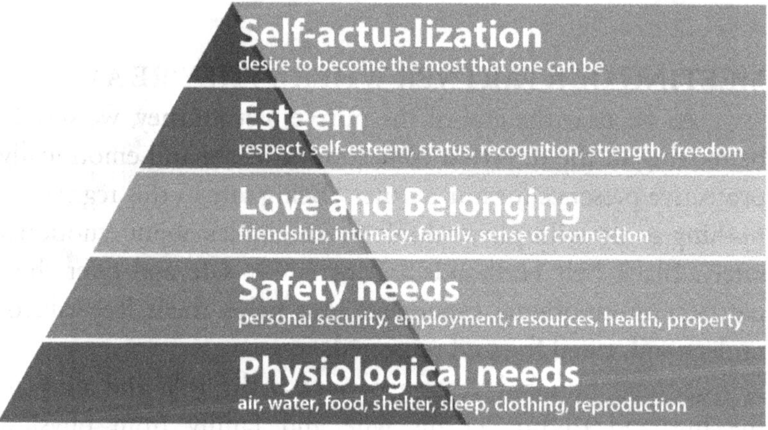
Self-actualization
desire to become the most that one can be
Esteem
respect, self-esteem, status, recognition, strength, freedom
Love and Belonging
friendship, intimacy, family, sense of connection
Safety needs
personal security, employment, resources, health, property
Physiological needs
air, water, food, shelter, sleep, clothing, reproduction

Looking at the depiction above, the plight of the 21st century marriage is this: Most men are excellent at providing for physiological needs and safety needs, but women are yearning for love & belonging needs and esteem needs. And this is the great disconnect of the modern marriage.

When we talk about creating a sense of emotional safety for our partners, we mean helping our spouses reach and fulfill higher level needs such as the love and belonging or esteem portions of the hierarchy of needs. Emotional safety in this context is about helping our wives feel valued, understood, cared for, and connected to us. This is what enables our partners to achieve higher level needs and to move beyond more basic and primitive needs. To bring the purple belt journey to fruition, we need to learn skills like being a good listener, not being a fixer, and learning how to share our emotions with our partner. These skills create the kind of emotional safety that woman crave, and help each of the two people in the relationship progress up the hierarchy of needs.

The reason emotional safety is placed at the end of purple belt work and not white belt work or blue belt work is because we first have to be very good at taking care of ourselves before we can focus on being emotionally available for our partners. We can't partner from an empty cup. We need to first fill our own cup, so we have something to offer our partners from our abundance. Too many men get this backwards; they feel compelled to try and offer their partners an emotionally connecting experience, but do it resentfully or half-heartedly because they don't experience the fulfillment of their own needs. True sacrifice will only be genuine and successful to the extent that we are prioritizing our needs as well.

"NO ONE IS GOING TO HURT YOU HERE"

Women are craving and yearning for a relationship with a man that offers them an opportunity to reach higher level needs. The truth is, so are all of us guys. This isn't a gender issue. I've never met a guy that wouldn't want to feel more cared for, respected, understood, and cherished. Any of us would.

Emotional safety isn't a complex idea and there's no reason to overcomplicate it. We can simply think of it as the building blocks that help us feel great about being in our relationship. It's the stuff that helps people *feel* in love.

If you're married and you're struggling financially to make ends meet, your first priority is to offer your wife a sense of physical safety through financial security. This will help her satisfy incredibly important, lower level needs. These critical lower level needs will take precedence over the emotional component that we're discussing in this chapter. Remember, the hierarchy of needs is a progression moving from lower level needs to higher level needs. We can't move to higher level needs until lower level needs are met. But for the majority of you reading this book, you're likely not living in poverty and wondering if you can put food on the table. Therefore, it's important to realize that lower level needs have likely been satisfied. Your next task is to offer your wife higher level needs. She's waiting for it. And it's an incredible gift to you too.

When we become more emotionally connected to our partners, we're divorce proofing our relationship and creating an environment that is rich with good feelings that no one would want to give it up. When we're emotionally connected, everyone wins, including us men. But so few men get this part right. They're still focused on lower level needs.

I've worked with hundreds of women who have initiated a divorce and after asking all of them why they left their marriages, here are some common themes that continually show up:

- "I feel terribly alone"
- "He only pays attention to me if he wants sex"
- "He never wants to listen to me"
- "He shoots down my dreams and ambitions"
- "He never opens up with me"
- "He feels like a stranger to me"

In the twenty-first century, most women are educated, capable of earning good money, and can provide for themselves in ways that meet their basic physiological and safety needs. Yet so many men see their primary function in marriage as one of meeting these lower level needs. One way men do this is by disproportionately focusing on generating greater levels of income, which is satisfying lower level needs. Women almost never leave a relationship because of financial reasons. In fact, I've never met one woman from the divorced couples I know who left for reasons related to money. Yet, if you dissect many marriages, you'd see how hard so many men work to be income providers. Which by itself is not bad. These are not bad men, they are in fact very good men, but they are simply shooting at the wrong target as to the nature of their role in their marriage.

Don't get me wrong, making money for your family is awesome. But not at the expense of providing higher level needs.

Women leave relationships for the bulleted reasons above – all of which happen to be emotional in nature. Women are leaving relationships because they don't feel emotionally connected, not because they fear their husbands can't care for them physically or financially. And not surprisingly, the same neglect of higher level needs are the reasons why men initiate divorce too.

Women, by and large in the twenty-first century, are looking to satisfy higher level needs from their husbands, and it's our job to learn the skills to be able to meet them there. As long as one person is asking for X, and one person is responding with Y, there will be a big disconnect. Our journey in becoming Black Belt Husband is to rise with the tide of being able to meet our partners wherever they reside on their own personal hierarchy of needs. This takes a little work on our part and might require us to learn a new skill or two, but it's worth it and the success of our relationships depends on it.

We have to get this right.

When I first started training Jiu-jitsu I was like most beginners in that I was a total spaz. There's something about BJJ that is unlike any other sport in that it can trigger some primal fight or flight aspects of ourselves because the essence of the sport is two people trying to choke each other unconscious. When you're new to the sport, it's common to be in a perpetual state of sheer panic. It's also what makes the sport so exhilarating. White Belts in BJJ flail and flop and do anything possible to *stay alive*. It happens to most who are starting and I was no exception.

One day shortly after beginning the sport, I was training with a very competent purple belt who was totally dominating me. As expected when a purple belt trains with a white belt, he submitted me about five times in five minutes. I was continually tapping to avoid being put to sleep. He was very good and I wasn't. As usual, I was spazzing all over the place. In that fight or flight panic state. When we were done training, he pulled me aside to a quiet space, looked me in the eyes and said, "Quentin, no one is going to hurt you here".

It was a profound moment for me and his words penetrated something deep in me. After he said that to me, I felt a mountain of emotions inside and I worked hard to hide the tears welling up in my eyes. You see, I came from a chaotic childhood where I did fear for my life on many occasions growing up with an alcoholic stepfather. I never knew if I was safe or not. In this moment, this purple belt was trying to tell me I didn't have to work so hard to fight for my life. He reminded me that I was safe. He was honoring his own development as a purple belt to care for a beginner white belt, and it was a pivotal moment in my BJJ training that allowed me to realize that I was safe among people who cared for me. I didn't need to fight for my life. We are trying to communicate the same emotional message to our wives: "No one is going to hurt you here".

AFFAIR-PROOFING YOUR MARRIAGE IS ABOUT EMOTIONAL SAFETY

The major contributing factor behind nearly all divorce is an inability on the part of one or both parties to offer their partner the basics to satiate the love and belonging or esteem needs. Instead they are continually offering their partner lower level needs that have already been met and satiated. When the denial of helping our partners reach higher level needs exists for too long, it creates an environment in marriage that is ripe for an affair.

Affairs, although a massively irresponsible way of dealing with any marital problems, are always a symptom of other underlying issues. People in happy marriages don't have affairs. It's that simple. Although affairs can be easily, but wrongly, looked at through the lens of being about sex, affairs are never really about sex. Affairs are always rooted in trying to satisfy a deeper emotional need and sex is never what people are truly looking for when they head down the road of infidelity. This is even true about one-night stands. When you talk with people who have worked through an affair, they will always tell you that the affair started because they felt disconnected, lonely, unimportant, and emotionally dissatisfied. Higher level needs being unmet. The actual sex part of an affair is just a derivative of satisfying emotional needs. All affairs are emotional affairs at their roots.

When we neglect to see the importance or relevance in creating an environment of emotional fulfillment in our relationships, an affair is always an inherent risk, no matter how moral or full of integrity someone believes themselves to be. Emotional needs are as important to relationships as a glass of water for the parched man walking across the desert. When we offer our partners more emotional support by listening well, attuning to their world, and being present, we are walking the path of the Black Belt Husband and accomplishing the journey through purple belt. Now that we have a solid foundation from our work on white and blue belts, we can offer our partners this higher level love they crave. This is what it means to affair-proof our marriage. We are not only hedging against our partners cheating, but we're also hedging against our own temptation to cheat.

DOMINATING OTHERS IS COWARDICE. CREATING SAFETY IS MASCULINE

A lot of guys get frustrated at the thought of being emotionally safe for their partners. Part of their frustration arises because a lot of wives do a horrible job being able to articulate their needs, which can make this process confusing. And part of their frustration comes from not feeling appreciated for what they do right. Many men hear the conversation about becoming more emotionally engaged with their partners as an accusation that they are deficient as husbands. Instead of seeing it this way, Black Belt Husbands view their need to be emotionally safe as a compliment to their success in satisfying lower level needs. They have been afforded the opportunity to offer their wives an even greater experience of life. I imagine you too have done a marvelous job creating a sense of security within your family through financial stability and congratulations for that! Now that you've done great in that department, you can move onward and upward. That's a compliment to you.

Black Belt Husbands understand the difference between offering their partners lower and higher-level needs. They recognize that if marriage is going to work successfully in the 21st century, satisfying higher level needs is a must. Black Belt Husbands care about their partners in a way that reflects their immense value as human beings and are willing to communicate their care by offering higher level needs. Our wives, and the mothers to our children deserve this type of care and respect from us. Black Belt Husbands see their spouses this way and have developed a skillset around emotional safety to the point where it comes easy.

In Brazilian Jiu-jitsu, everyone understands the danger of training with white belts. Their carelessness and lack of skill causes them to act in ways that are dangerous to their training partners. Since white belts don't have the experience, the necessary fundamentals, or body awareness, they put their partners at a higher risk for injury than higher ranking belts. Black belts in BJJ by contrast don't have the same reputation. If you train with a black belt in BJJ, you're never worried about getting accidently and carelessly injured. They are controlled and tempered. The irony is that their extreme competence makes them the safest. Even though BJJ black belts are master assassins, they are the safest ones in the gym. That's the irony: the most skilled are the most safe, and the least skilled are the most dangerous.

In marriage, it's the same way. Black Belt Husbands are the safest because they have a skillset and level of competence in marriage that gives their partners an experience of safety, and not injury.

The wives of Black Belt Husbands feel protected, emotionally safe, and cared for.

To offer your partner this experience from a place of strength is a true sign of masculine integrity. A BJJ Black Belt and Black Belt Husband are both positions that come with great responsibility. They both demand that each title creates a sense of safety for those amidst their care. In BJJ, black belts offer a sense of physical safety and Black Belt Husbands offer a sense of emotional safety. Both are true expressions of authentic masculinity.

THIS IS NOT YOUR FATHER'S MARRIAGE

Most of us didn't grow up with fathers who role modeled the experience of emotional safety. That doesn't mean your dad was a bad dad or a bad husband to your mom. Concepts of emotional safety weren't on the radar in past generations to the extent they are today. Husbands in prior generations, for the most part, were rewarded for satisfying lower level needs. This is why the idea of being a solid financial provider as a husband has carried so much weight historically and still is part of the paradigm for so many men today. It was the most important thing in prior generations. However, generally speaking, since the 1960's most women have been able to provide for themselves financially and aren't looking exclusively for financial security from a partner. The reason this matters is because we learn almost everything about marriage from our parents. And the truth is, being emotionally safe simply wasn't as critical in the past as it is today. Many men today don't see the need to be emotionally available because they didn't see their fathers do it. So many of us are learning what being emotionally safe means for the first time as adults. How would you rate your own level of emotional safety with your partner? Knowing that your wife needs you to provide for higher level needs, where do you think you stack up?

- What do you think about sharing your own emotions with your wife? Particularly more vulnerable feelings? Do you have a stigma in your mind that sharing your feelings is a sign of being less manly? That's a common thought for many men, so don't feel bad if you've ever felt that way. It's something with which I still struggle.
- Would you describe your dad as being emotionally available? Did he share his feelings with your mom? Was he a good listener? Or was he more of a problem solver and a fixer? Again, this is not a criticism of your dad, we're just trying to understand where we come from.
- Speaking of fixers, have you ever been accused of being a fixer? Usually, fixer's are guys who have a hard time with listening well and rush quickly toward problem solving. How would you rate yourself in this area?

- To be a good listener, it actually takes a little work. You have to pay attention to body language, tone, facial expression, emotion, and lastly, the words. When it comes to listening to your wife, do you think you're really hearing her?
- Empathy is a cornerstone of being emotionally safe. How would you rate your skillset with being empathic with your partner?
- How well do you do with providing emotional safety and connection for your partner when she is going through a tough time? And are you able to share with her when you're going through a tough time?

These questions can get you started thinking about how you may stack up with the concept of being an emotionally safe presence for your partner. Being emotionally safe is high ranking purple belt stuff because your ability to do it really separates you from most men. In my assessment, I would say that roughly 10 percent of men have an adequate skill set when it comes to being emotionally safe. If this is something you struggle with, don't feel bad. You can learn how to do it all.

BLACK BELT HUSBAND TRAINING: LEARNING TO SPEAK A NEW LANGUAGE

Purple Belts in BJJ are very competent practitioners of their craft. By the time someone trains BJJ consistently for six years or more and earns a purple belt, they know very well what they are doing. Since we're rounding the corner with finishing our purple belt on our way toward Black Belt Husband, there is also an expectation that by this point you are also competent in your craft as a husband. It doesn't mean that you can't make mistakes, but it does mean that you shouldn't be making white belt mistakes. Being arrogant, defensive, and passive aggressive, etc. are lower belt mistakes. I'm assuming by the time you're finishing up your purple belt, you've got that stuff sorted out. At the very least, you should be able to catch yourself quickly. You're getting ready to earn your brown belt and mastering emotional safety is an essential step you can't miss if you're to move forward. Learning how to be emotionally safe can be difficult in and of itself. You don't need to spend any energy on white belt mistakes at this point.

Creating an environment of emotional safety helps our partners feel more connected to us and us to them. Emotional safety is the bonding agent that glues two people together and solidifies their connection in relationship. Being emotionally safe is one of the key differentiators that separates average dissatisfied husbands and Black Belt Husbands. Generally speaking, there are two foundational elements at the heart of developing emotional safety. To keep it simple, we'll talk about these elements as giving and receiving.

GIVING EMOTIONALLY (The first half of emotional safety)

When we think about giving emotionally, we're talking about how well we share ourselves with the ones we love. Our partners get to know us and feel close to us when we share our emotional worlds with them. Without the process of sharing, how is anybody supposed to *really* know us or understand us? They simply can't. Our partners can only know a slim and shallow portion of us if we discount the critical need to share more about who we really are, emotionally.

Many guys struggle with this aspect of sharing emotionally because they fear their wives will see them as weak or less manly. Other guys worry that their partners can't be there for them or that they don't care about their feelings. Still others think so wrongly that they don't have feelings all together. Whatever might keep you from opening up to your partner or your band of brothers, it's essential that you tackle the issue. We have to be able to share ourselves with our loved ones. A relationship without sharing will be shallow, empty, and eventually die a slow death from disconnection. A very simple, and practical way to begin moving in a new and healthy direction is to commit to sharing just one emotion with your partner every day. Sometimes, it's just a matter of getting more comfortable with doing it regularly until you realize that it's not as weird and scary as you imagined. It looks something like this:

"Today, when I was _______________, I felt _______________, and was thinking ___________________ _______________."

It's really that simple, there's no need to overcomplicate it. The more you do it with regularity and consistency, the more your partner will get to know you better and feel closer to you. All good stuff. All higher level stuff.

RECEIVING EMOTIONALLY (The second half of emotional safety)

The second half of the emotional safety equation is about learning how to be a good receiver of emotions, which requires that we listen well. Being a good listener, or active listener is magic for any relationship. Without it, the relationship will feel hopelessly frustrating. Listening well is an active process. It requires that we put ourselves into a mindset of being present, attentive, and engaged. Being an active listener involves three simple steps: mirroring, validating, and empathizing.

Step One: Mirroring - Mirroring consists of making a simple statement while you're actively listening to your partner that shows you're paying close attention to what they're saying. Say you're talking to your partner and she says, "I'm feeling so frustrated at those other parents at Johnny's soccer game!" A mirroring response looks something like this: "So, you're feeling frustrated at those other parents - what happened?" Mirroring means echoing back what you heard, in your own words, to help your partner confidently know that you are tracking with them.

Step Two: Validating – When you validate, you let your partner know she's not crazy for feeling how she feels. Validating looks something like this: Your wife says, "At the soccer game the other parents were being so rude to the referee, it was so frustrating". A validating response looks like, "That's totally understandable you would be frustrated, I might be frustrated too". To validate someone, you're simply trying to let them know that you're paying attention to the feelings in their message. To validate well, you don't have to agree with your partner. You're simply trying to connect with them.

Step Three: Empathizing - Empathizing, the last step in the actively listening process, is about letting your partner know you care about their feelings. Here's how it works; Your wife says, "It was so frustrating watching the other parents act so ridiculous!" An empathic response is something like, "I'm really sorry you were so frustrated during the game and that you had to see all of that". Metaphorically speaking, empathy is a process of stepping inside the mind of your partner and trying to relate to how she feels. Again, you're not agreeing or disagreeing; if you get lost in disagreement, you've veered way off course. When it comes to empathizing, you can't disagree with someone's subjective emotional experience. You can only empathize with it.

Developing our ability to give and receive emotionally is a critical part of rounding out the purple belt journey. Many of us are simply not used to talking or listening this way; when we try it, we might feel a bit awkward or uncomfortable. The experience is similar to learning a new language. Though we may stumble through it at first, with practice, we'll become fluent. After a certain point, we won't even need to think about it. I applaud all of you men who are willing to push through your own discomfort and stretch yourselves to become more well-rounded and multidimensional. It isn't easy, and I applaud your bravery and willingness to challenge yourself. You're on your way to Black Belt Husband.

FOR HER, EMOTIONAL SAFETY EQUATES TO TRUST

Becoming an emotionally safe presence for your partner is going to pay huge dividends. When we learn how to be emotionally safe, we may notice all sorts of things begin to shift in our relationship. We fight less, have more sex, and our wives respecting us more. When our partners begin to feel more connected to us emotionally, everything in the relationship flows more easily. When people are satisfying higher level needs, they're just a lot happier. Growing in emotional safety is not a small tweak, but a total transformative opportunity to make everything better.

Offering your partner an emotionally safe experience in the relationship also contributes to divorce-proofing your relationship. The lack of emotional safety is the reason why women leave marriages. They don't leave to find better men, they leave to find more emotionally available men. 70 percent of divorces are initiated by women and the overwhelming reason they leave is in search of higher level needs. We could judge women's decisions to leave a marriage as wrong or immoral, but at the end of the day we have to take responsibility for ourselves and perhaps our limitations in this area. If emotional safety is lacking in the marriage, everything is at risk. It matters that much.

So often I hear husbands talk about how they feel disrespected by their wives. Their wives aggressively challenge them, demean them, or relentlessly critique or question their decisions. Of course, this drives men crazy and husbands often feel totally hopeless about it. But here's what I've noticed in all of the relationships I've seen; I've never met a wife who was disrespectful to her husband when she felt emotionally safe. Feelings of emotional unsafety are always behind the apparent disrespect. I'm not advocating that her being disrespectful is good or a healthy response to her feeling emotionally unsafe. But I want you to see the root of where this comes from within her. Your wife may critique you, challenge you, and demean you because she doesn't trust you, emotionally. Trust for her is earned by helping her feel emotionally safe. The answer is helping her feel emotionally safe. We have to give to get, and if you pride yourself on being a leader, give first and learn how to give the right things. Give her the emotional safety she's craving and her interactions with you will change.

PURPLE BELT SKILLS TEST

PRACTICAL SKILL NEEDED TO MOVE FORWARD

To graduate from purple belt and move on toward Black Belt Husband, we have to develop our skillset in being more emotionally safe. To do this, we need a baseline understanding of emotions and the purpose they serve for our wives. As Black Belt Husbands, we're getting to the root of her feelings.

Required Skill: Thirty Days to Break Through Her Criticism

Spending time with someone who relentlessly criticizes can be frustrating and draining. The negativity and nagging can make many people question their sanity. But why do so many women interact this way with their husbands?

Well, here's what we need to know. Your wife communicates her deeper, more vulnerable feelings through criticism. Said another way, when your wife criticizes you, she's expressing that she doesn't feel emotionally safe. More specifically, she doesn't feel safe enough to communicate her more authentic and vulnerable feelings like sadness, hurt, or fear. Think of criticism as her defense mechanism against vulnerable feelings.

Over the next thirty days, I want you to keep a journal of every time your partner nags you, criticizes you, or tries to control you. Every time you journal about an incident, think about what she might be feeling. To keep it simple, use the top three vulnerable feelings; sadness, hurt, or fear. As you keep your running journal, you'll notice themes and patterns for your wife that point to a deeper, more vulnerable feeling. As you get clear in your own mind about what her criticism expresses (either hurt, sadness, or fear) you can begin asking her about these deeper, more authentic, and vulnerable feelings. As the two of you begin to open up conversations about these feelings, you'll be making huge deposits into the emotional safety piggy-bank, which will reward you greatly.

PURPLE BELT ATTRIBUTES SUMMARY

Before we move on to brown belt, let's recap what we've learned in purple belt. The purple belt journey is all about becoming well-rounded and mastering the finer points of becoming a Black Belt Husband. As we move toward Black Belt Husband, the purple belt work has us focusing on becoming more playful in our interactions, building a band of brothers, and realizing the importance of offering our partners a sense of safety through emotional availability. The purple belt experience is about sharpening our swords. Let's recap what we've learned in the purple belt journey.

Purple Belt I—Playful Summary:

Life has become much too serious for many husbands. Overworked and stressed out, the average husband is miserable to be around. But this is not how your relationship began. In the beginning, you were fun, playful, and you offered your partner a sense of excitement and joy. Of course, there are times when you need to be serious and steadfast, but that shouldn't be the norm most of the time. If you are playful with her, it will invigorate her joy toward you.

Purple Belt II—Connected Summary:

When you try to navigate the marriage journey isolated from other men that share similar values as you, you're destined to veer off course. You need a band of brothers to keep you accountable and with whom you can share the experiences of marriage. Your band of brothers gives you support, friendship, accountability, and alignment with your core values. Self-reliance has its value in the right context, but it's also the marriage Achilles heel for many men who live disconnected from other men.

Purple Belt III—Safe Summary:

Becoming emotionally safe in your marriage divorce proofs your relationship. This wasn't as critical to the success of marriage for past generations as it is today. Becoming emotionally safe is offering her *protection* from a 21st century standpoint and helping her reach higher level needs. Being emotionally safe isn't just for your wife's benefit. You have much to gain too. Emotional safety is the glue that not only holds the relationship together but makes it feel so good that you can't imagine life without it.

Congratulations!
You've graduated from Purple Belt!

SECTION FOUR

The Brown Belt Journey; Being a Leader Worth Following

Discipline and consistency. I owe these two factors for all I have attained in my life. Things have never happened overnight. Results have appeared as a consequence of decades long toil. It is necessary to persist.
—Master Carlos Gracie Jr., Founder of Gracie Barra Jiu-Jitsu

GETTING READY FOR THE BROWN BELT JOURNEY

The brown belt journey is all about creating an environment of natural leadership in marriage. But being a good leader is hard and the privilege of leading is only earned, never given. Before we arrive at Black Belt Husband, we're going to talk about three important attributes that make us leaders in marriage: being intentionally other-centered, developing a strong sense of loyalty, and being purposeful in our mission. When these three qualities are layered on top of our white belt, blue belt, and purple belt work, we become magnetizing leaders who our partners easily follow.

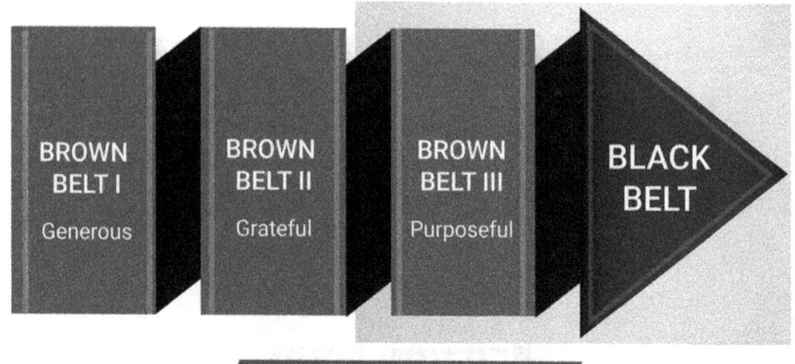

CHAPTER 10
Brown Belt I:
Generous; Leading by Other-Centeredness

SHIFTING FROM ME-CENTERED TO OTHER-CENTERED

The brown belt journey is about honing leadership skills in marriage. To begin this journey, we need to reevaluate our ability to move from a me-centered marriage to a generous other-centered marriage.

Being generously other-centered is a foundational quality of true leadership. Great leaders have one thing in common: the people who follow them truly believe that they have their best interest in mind. They are generously other-centered. Being generously other-centered isn't an optional part of the Black Belt Husband process and the brown belt stopover is about exploring this aspect of being a great husband. We can't be the kinds of husbands that our wives brag about until we become more other-centered.

The road thus far to brown belt has been about shoring up our own resources and reclaiming our internal strength so that we can become appropriately and generously other-centered in our marriage. Now that we are stronger and more self-confident, we can afford the emotional expenditures of giving to others. People who struggle with being other-centered aren't selfish, usually it is because they have an empty cup and don't have anything to offer. Being other-centered is about true and authentic sacrifice, not a cheap cliché that gets loosely thrown around.

True sacrifice can only be done from a place of strength. If we sacrifice from a place of weakness or fear, it's an unhealthy version of codependency. Marriage help books talk endlessly about the need to sacrifice, but they often miss that strength always precedes sacrifice. If our cup is empty, we can't give anyone water, no matter how much we may try. Many marriages have gone awry because men have thought that sacrifice was the right thing to do, but they did it out of fear or deprivation. This always leads to a mountain of resentment.

The irony is that the more we give to ourselves by taking good care of ourselves and appropriately asserting our needs, the more we can give to others from a place of strength without any resentment. The Black Belt Husband is generously other-centered, not because he can't be me-centered, but because he has enough strength and inner-completeness to choose to be generously other-centered.

BEING OTHER-CENTERED MAKES YOU A LEADER WORTH FOLLOWING

There are moments in every relationship when the people involved have competing needs. You want this, and she wants that. The unwillingness to relent in these scenarios is not an attribute of Black Belt Husbands. Other-centered communicates to your wife and your family that you are making the choice to do so. The key word here is choice.

When we choose to be other-centered instead of me-centered, we're being self-aware and deliberate. We also can choose to make me-centered decisions, but we never make these decisions from a place of insecurity. As brown belts nearing the rank of Black Belt Husband, all of our choices must be deliberate. They cannot be driven by fears of conflict, disappointing others, or feelings of shame.

When we choose to say yes knowing we could just as easily say no, we're being generous from a place of strength.

This is what it means to be a leader in marriage. When you begin the brown belt journey, the expectation is that you're prepared for more other-centeredness. You're choosing to be other-centered out of a place of genuine care and concern. Your cup is full and you can offer to others.

In BJJ we see this principle playing out clearly by the time people get their brown belts. Brown belts in BJJ are often running classes, coaching others, and are looked upon by lower ranking students as the teacher. When brown belts in BJJ teach, they are graciously and gratefully giving back what they have been given. Paying it forward is a fundamental tenant in BJJ. If BJJ brown belts didn't help the newer students, fewer people would learn the art and enjoy the experience. Brown belts could smash everyone with whom they trained, but it wouldn't be in alignment with the spirit of BJJ. The same holds true for brown belts in the Black Belt Husband journey. At this point, we're not engaging in petty squabbles about silly things, holding grudges, or storming off when we don't get our way. We're challenging ourselves to be leaders worth following.

ME-CENTERED LEADERSHIP LEADS TO HORRIBLE POWER STRUGGLES

Some men have unhelpful ideas about what it means to be a leader in their marriage. When they use the term leader, some men are referring to an authoritarian figure who has ultimate control in the relationship and can't be questioned. I suppose this is a type of leadership, but it's not an effective way of doing things in a twenty-first century marriage or business. As leadership principles have expanded in business, so too have leadership principles changed in marriage. Authoritarian bosses may still work for the low-wage factory worker, but do you see your wife as the low-wage factory worker? Business publications continue to report how successful companies are able to retain their employees better than other companies. More often than not, other-centered leadership is the one thing that is responsible more than any other thing for employee retention.

When a husband doesn't have enough other-centeredness in marriage, the couple will likely get stuck in a nasty power struggle. Each person either overtly or covertly tries to assert their power. When this goes on long enough, it erodes any sense of stability or trust in the relationship. Each person, over time, begins to see the other as someone who is trying to take from them instead of someone who is trying to give to them. The end results aren't pretty.

Becoming a Black Belt Husband is about shattering the me-centeredness that creates power struggles in marriage. Black Belt Husbands are strong enough that they can give plenty and feel confident that they'll get enough. When we sacrifice our own wants and needs from a place of fullness and strength, we earn respect and admiration from our partners. The respect and admiration we receive from being great leaders nearly always translates to more peace and harmony in the marriage and forever are gone the horrible power struggles.

THE ONLY SACRIFICE THAT COUNTS IS SACRIFICE DONE OUT OF STRENGTH

Becoming generously other-centered from a place of strength is a signpost of the mature masculine. The generosity that is rooted in strength is a time-tested attribute of the greatest men of history. Battle-tested generals, CEO's, and NBA coaches have one thing in common: other-centeredness.

By contrast, immature men who have not developed their full masculine potential, relish the feeling of power that comes from being a leader. It's like a hit of a drug and they want more of it because the rush they feel when they are in the dominant position and have control. But the need to be in a controlling dominant position is a childish need, and mature masculine men feel strong enough within themselves to relinquish that need. I sadly and embarrassingly spent many years vacillating back and forth between feeling the need to be in charge, and cowering under passivity and fear based compliance. It's such a burden to live this way. But how could I know any other way? This is what I was taught to do. Both sides of the continuum are an emotional death sentence, and neither sides are Black Belt Husband material. With time, I've come to realize that there is a better way.

The mature masculine leader wants to see others make a more meaningful life for themselves. Psychological profiles are nearly always a given for potential leadership candidates in order to identify this capacity. Good leaders are always other-centered and concerned for the collective group more than their me-centered egos. But they are also very confident and self-assure as well. Other-centered and confident are the two complimentary qualities for the successful leader in Black Belt Husband

When we become other-centered in our homes, we're role-modeling what true strength looks like for the little boys and little girls watching us closely. When we act controlling in the name of leadership, or fearfully passive in the name of "sacrifice", our children may be watching and adopting similar patterns for later life. Becoming more other-centered is not for the faint of heart. If it was easy, power struggles wouldn't be such a common and destructive force in the average marriage. But Black Belt Husbands are not average. We're the very few mature masculine men who can honestly give to our spouses from a place of strength.

HOW WOULD YOU RATE YOUR OWN LEVEL OF OTHER-CENTEREDNESS?

How would you evaluate your level of generous other-centeredness in your relationship? Are you operating like a sacrificial leader? Are you giving from a place of strength and confidence or are you sacrificing as a way to avoid conflict? Are you genuinely concerned about those who follow you, to the point where you'll set aside your own wants and needs, or does being in control feel good to you? Being genuinely other-centered is about feeling confident enough to set aside your own needs for the success and betterment of those you care about. Take some time and journal about these questions to get a sense of where you're at as a generous other-centered leader.

- Being a good leader requires that you build trust for those that follow you. How has trust been compromised in your relationship?
- What have you learned from your father about leadership in marriage and do you think his strategies would be successful if implemented today? Historically, leadership in marriage either looked patriarchal or matriarchal. Are you able to create a more egalitarian form of leadership in your home?
- Even better, can you create so much trust and safety that your wife prefers to follow your lead?
- How are you at creating win-win scenarios for dilemmas in your marriage?
- The work you've done to get to this point has been about building enough strength and confidence to be able to lead confidently other-centered. Too many men try to be leaders too soon without the required strength, only to resent their spouse for their "sacrifice". Are you ready to lead by other-centeredness or do you need more time to get stronger? There's no shame in needing more time.

- Other-centeredness shifts the focus from "me" to "her" in a way that's impossible to miss. If you were to ask your wife whether she thinks you are more me-centered, or other-centered, what do you think she would say?

EFFECTIVE LEADERS ASK GREAT OTHER-CENTERED QUESTIONS

Becoming more generously other-centered begins with enough self-confidence and internal strength to set aside our needs for the needs of someone we care about. For some who arrive at this chapter and struggle with being generously other-centered, it's often because there isn't a solid foundation of internal strength and self-confidence. If we're in this position, we may need to revisit some concepts of the blue belt work to get a better handle on being more honest and assertive. If we find it difficult to be a sacrificial leader and we end up in petty power struggles, there's a good chance that we need to spend some more time being honest, assertive, and getting more comfortable with the conflict that usually ensues. In this case, please don't hesitate to revisit the work in blue belt.

However, if we feel we're ready to employ more sacrificial leadership strategies, one easy and very effective way to do it is with great questions. The simple act of asking a good question of your wife powerfully communicates that you care enough to slow down, pause, set aside your own needs, and engage them. This kind of engagement is part of being a great leader. Great leaders remain actively engaged and genuinely curious about the people they lead, which demonstrates their other-centeredness. In order to develop our other-centeredness muscle, we must begin by proactively engaging with our partners in more other-centered ways.

Have you ever worked for a boss who took little interest in getting to know who you were? I have, and it's always unfulfilling. By contrast, I've also worked for leaders that went out of their way to get to know me. They asked me questions about my family, my interests, and how I was doing. I knew intuitively that these leaders genuinely cared about me because of their intentional other-centeredness. They didn't have to go out of their way to engage me, but they chose the path of other-centeredness. After all, I got a paycheck, so wasn't that enough? As a result, I always gave my best to them. To become Black Belt Husbands, we're going to engage our wives in a similar way.

Too often, us guys, are running at a million miles per hour and we forget to slow down long enough to ask the people we care about how they are really doing. This is a sign of an ineffective leader; too busy frantically focused on his own needs that he forgets to check on his people. We don't want to make the same mistake at home. Great leaders at home slow down long enough, set aside their own busy schedules, and actively engage their spouses. They do it because they genuinely care and they know the enormous benefit this provides. These interactions build safety and trust, which allows her to feel good about following you.

Here is a list of simple and powerful questions that you can use to begin actively engaging your wife to foster more other-centeredness. Use these questions to open up a dialogue about her life. You'll be surprised by what you learn and even more surprised by how much she appreciates it. Your willingness to be other-centered will inspire her to follow you as she begins to trust you. The secret in it all is that you have to be still and present when you ask these questions. You can't be rushing out the door, on your phone checking email, or distracted with something on the television. When you ask, you have to care enough to pay attention to the answer. If you're distracted, don't ask. Wait for a better time when you're more present and can really take in her answer.

BLACK BELT HUSBAND TRAINING: ENGAGING HER WITH OTHER-CENTEREDNESS

Easy Everyday Questions:

Below you'll find questions that you can use to initiate conversations with your wife on a daily basis. These are questions that you can use over and over again; she'll never get tired of answering them. People love being asked about their day and how they're doing. It's really simple. The questions don't need to be complex or overwhelming. When asked with genuine curiosity, they will clearly communicate to your wife that you are stepping outside yourself and generously stepping inside her world. It's a gesture that will help her to feel safe enough to follow your lead.

- What was the best part of your day today?
- What was the worst part of your day today?
- Did I do anything that hurt you today?
- Is there anything I can do for you to make your life easier?
- How would you like to spend more meaningful time together?
- Is there anything I can do that would make you feel more cared for?

Easy In-Depth Questions:

These questions are dream questions that you can use from time to time to communicate your other-centeredness in a more unique way outside of everyday life questions. They are the questions you used to ask when you were first dating your wife, but likely stopped asking over time. It's likely that the answers to these questions for her are different today than they were when you first were dating. Asking involved questions in a spirit of other-centeredness is a sign of leading well in marriage.

A word of caution:

These questions are great, but they are analogous to working out intensely once a month and neglecting physical activity the other twenty-nine days. Great relationships are similar to great physical health in that they're about the small victories matched with unwavering consistency. Brown belts in marriage, like brown belts in Jiu-jitsu train several times a week, perfecting their craft. Use these questions as an adjunct to support the more routine "everyday" questions listed above.

- If this year was a success, what would be different for you at the end of the year?
- If you were given a million dollars, how would you spend the money?
- What do you want to be known most for at the end of your life?
- What's one hobby or skill that you've wanted to learn, but never got the chance?
- What are you most proud of in your life right now?
- How have you been feeling about us lately?
- Do you have any regrets about your life that you wish you could take back?
- Are you satisfied with our mutual goals or would you like them to be different?
- Where would you like to travel to if you could go anywhere tomorrow?
- What aspects of my personality do you love and what aspects do you wish were different?

THE IRONY OF GETTING A LOT BY GIVING A LOT

When we become more other-centered in marriage, it opens up a whole new world of good feelings. Being generously other-centered is the way out of those horrible power struggles that never lead anywhere. Being more other-centered communicates to your wife that you genuinely care about her success and want to see her fulfilled. When she feels this energy from you, she naturally sees you as someone who's on her side and giving to her, as opposed to someone who takes from her. In other words, she will begin to see you as a leader she wants to follow.

All of us need leaders to follow. I do, you do, and so do our wives. Our lives at home provide us opportunities to be sacrificial leaders that help our partners feel safe, trusting, and cared for. Being other-centered moves us out of authoritarian styles of relating to more collaborative styles that are inclusive and revolve around win-win solutions. However, we can only be sacrificial leaders to the extent that we feel enough self-confidence and self-assuredness within ourselves. Without this, we will resent the feeling of having to give. Ironically, the more we give in marriage from a place of strength, the more we get. When we see marriage as an opportunity to be other-centered, we end up being the big winners and beneficiaries because our wives naturally adopt the other-centered mindset as well. Imagine a scenario where two people are trying to outbid each other with other-centeredness instead of two people trying to outbid each other with me-centeredness. That's what we're working toward.

When you're intentionally other-centered with your partner, a whole new world of relationship excitement begins to open up. Instead of feeling bogged down, angry, and stuck in the power struggle of "what about me?", you begin to feel relaxed. The feeling is often similar to how couples felt when they first started dating. As you intentionally work toward maintaining your other-centeredness, something miraculous happens; your wife begins to feel more connected to you. She will notice that you are much more present with her - something that nearly every woman wants more of from her man. As you become more present and generously other-centered, she's going to respond to you in ways you've most likely been wanting. The positive ripple effect toward you will pay huge dividends. You will find her kinder, more engaged, and most likely much more sexual with you. The benefits of leading with other-centeredness far outweigh the effort.

BROWN BELT SKILLS TEST

PRACTICAL SKILL NEEDED TO MOVE FORWARD

The road toward becoming a Black Belt Husband is paved with other-centeredness. When we're lower ranking belts, we don't expect ourselves to be generously giving to our partners. We were still at a place where we were learning how to advocate for our own needs. But as brown belts we need to see the importance of giving back and relishing in the success of others. As brown belts, we need to begin mentoring others in the marriage journey.

Required Skill: Commit to Mentoring a White Belt in Marriage

You have a lot to offer someone else. Others need your guidance and your coaching on how to be a great husband. Even if you don't feel like you have all the answers, you have more answers than many and that can be life changing. At this point in the journey, it's time to start giving back, not only to your wife, but to another husband. I want you to find a white belt husband somewhere in the world and mentor him on what it means to be a great husband. This is different than interacting with your band of brothers, all of whom are at a similar place in the journey. This is a one-directional relationship where you're helping someone else along the way. In BJJ, the process is just the same. I've never met a brown belt who wasn't simultaneously a teacher, a coach, and a leader. Now it's your turn to help another man who knows far less than you. You're ready for this.

CHAPTER 11

Brown Belt II:
Grateful; Appreciation That Cements Our Loyalty

LOYALTY IS A BYPRODUCT OF GRATITUDE

BJJ black belts are incredibly loyal to the schools where they've trained and have spent years perfecting their craft. But why is their loyalty to particular schools so strong? When someone receives a Black Belt in BJJ, it's usually a deeply emotional moment that is often filled with tears of joy. The hard work and toil required to get that far is an accomplishment that rivals any achievement in life. Without the training partners, the coaches, and the lineage of those who came before, the BJJ black belt would not have been able to arrive at such an enormous achievement. Black belts develop a deep appreciation for the experiences and the people who made it possible.

The gratitude they carry drives their undying loyalty.

Just as BJJ black belts are deeply loyal, so too are Black Belt Husbands. The kind of loyalty that Black Belts Husbands have in their relationship is a byproduct of the gratitude they have learned to foster and develop for what they have been given. Black Belt Husbands have a deep appreciation for their marriage and even all of the challenges that have provided them an opportunity to grow more fully as husbands.

By contrasts, white belts in BJJ are rarely loyal. BJJ white belts are notorious for hopping from school to school until they find the right fit. This is not a bad thing, and it's important that people find what's right for them, but as we're nearing the end of the Black Belt Husband journey, it's important to see the need for a deeper gratitude that drives our loyalty. We're rounding the brown belt corner and showing that we're leaders worth following. Great leaders are always loyal to their people.

In our life experiences, we always have the choice to see things with a sense of appreciation or with a sense of discontent. We can say, "I'm appreciative of this…", or we can say "I'm not thankful….". Everything in life can be viewed this way. When we aspire to become Black Belt Husbands, it's essential that we know how to be more grounded in a posture of gratitude. As we make progress, we see our lives and our experiences with our partners, and even the challenges we face from the perspective of, "I'm appreciative of this…". True gratitude and appreciation cement our loyalty; and without them, our sense of loyalty will always teeter and be subject to our shifting circumstances.

BEING GRATEFUL FOR WHAT WE HAVE, INSTEAD OF BITTER FOR WHAT WE DON'T

Being grounded in gratitude is an essential part of the Black Belt Husband journey. Without gratitude, we'll always see what is wrong and what needs to be different instead of seeing what we have to appreciate. Being grateful is not a delusional state of mind in which we deny difficulties or suppress our desires. Remember, during our blue belt work, we get stronger by learning how to be more open and honest about what's important to us. We're no longer afraid to share what really matters with our partners. But being honest about what is important to us, and being in a posture of gratitude are not mutually exclusive.

So, we can do both. We can be open and honest, and also be deeply appreciative of what we have. Husbands who have a hard time getting grounded in gratitude tend to perpetually see the bad in their partners. It's a pessimistic lens that clouds the relationship. Their thought life can be consumed with obsessing about how bad their partner is. All of us are susceptible to getting caught in these negative thought loops. If we do begin to see things this way, we need tools to step out of it and see things in a more balanced way.

There is a famous quote by Abraham Lincoln that says, "We can complain that rose bushes have thorns, or we can rejoice that thorn bushes have roses". Developing a posture of gratitude helps us see the inherent good in our partners. We can come to appreciate ever so greatly what we have when we adopt gratitude as a way of being. The big payoff for our relationships is that gratitude gives rise to more loyalty. Without gratitude, the relationship will always seem to be teetering on the edge of collapse because our attention is directed to what's wrong. And of course over time, we can build a great case about how wrong and bad it is in this frame of mind. Black Belt Husbands aren't seeing their relationships through this lens of discontent. A gratitude mindset stabilizes the relationship and cements our loyalty to it, which creates a great amount of security for everyone involved. Without gratitude, we vacillate back and forth about the relationship. The relationship feels like it hinges on the feelings of the moment. With deeper gratitude, we're steady and present.

BLACK BELT HUSBANDS UNDERSTAND THE GRASS IS NOT GREENER

I spent years of my living without much gratitude. I was always searching for the next best thing. I did it in romantic relationships, friendships, jobs, etc. and was certain there was something "better" out there for me. If things ever got tough in relationships, it was my instinct to think, "maybe this relationship is wrong". As a result, I bounced around from relationship to relationship, absolutely certain that the right one was just around the corner. One little rock of the boat and I was ready to jump ship and swim for the shore. I spent many years without the maturity it takes to see that the grass is not greener.

With maturity, we come to take notice and appreciate what we have, instead of wondering whether the grass is greener on the other side. This applies to all areas of our lives. When we're not appreciative, we tend to look for the thing that will fulfill us *out there*. But the truth is, that thing out there doesn't exist. It's an illusion that offers us a false promise. Fulfillment comes from within, not from the outside.

To illustrate the truth of this principle, we can look at the statistics on divorce rates for second and third marriages. Most people know that divorce rates for first marriages are around 50 percent, but what many don't know is that divorce rates for second marriages are around 70 percent, and divorce rates for third marriages are around 80 percent. Why does this matter? It speaks to the fact that leaving one marriage in hopes of finding the "right" partner doesn't exist - statistically speaking.

Online dating now affords single people the opportunity to choose among literally millions of potential candidates for a relationship. With such a large pool to choose from, we would surely be able to find the *right one*, right? But even amidst so many choices, we still can't find the right one, as evidenced by the divorce rate for second and third marriages. If it was about finding the right one, the divorce rate should decrease for second and third marriages, right? But it doesn't, and this data reminds us that the grass isn't greener, despite our fantasy that it will be so. Making relationships work isn't about finding the right one; it's about becoming the "right one".

MATURE MASCULINITY IS HONORABLY LOYAL

Loyalty and commitment are highly regarded virtues among mature masculine men. The gratitude that sustains loyalty and commitment in relationships is a highly honorable characteristic. It is *the way* of the mature masculine man. By contrast, young boys are less loyal and less committed; they get a free pass because they're just boys. Loyalty is a cornerstone virtue of Black Belt Husbands and this asset of personality separates Black Belt Husbands from the pack. Loyalty and commitment are disappearing virtues in our "what's-in-it-for-me", easily disposable modern world and this creates an undercurrent of deep insecurity in most marriages. But instead of just telling people to "be loyal", we want to develop the mindset and know how to build loyalty in our relationships. And we do that through gratitude.

Gratitude, loyalty, and commitment are the way of the Black Belt Husband. A lack of appreciation, pettiness, complaints, and a narrow me-focused attitude is white belt stuff. None of us will ever be satisfied in life and relationships with this frame of mind. Divorce rates for second and third marriages prove that happiness doesn't come from a new relationship or a "better partner". Unfortunately this is how most of the world understands how to be successful in relationships. But you're in a different camp - you're in the Black Belt Husband ten percent, which means you're going to harness a mindset around appreciation that is going to cement your loyalty. This is the way of the mature masculine man.

ARE YOU SEEING THORNS OR ROSE PETALS?

So how would you rate the level of gratitude you experience in your relationships and in your life? And how does your ability or inability to feel grateful influence the level of happiness, peace, loyalty and commitment that sustains your relationship? A happy and committed long-term relationship is not possible without lots of gratitude. But we often forget to focus on what is good in the relationship and instead get myopically focused on what is wrong. Take some time in solitude and read through the questions below to assess your own level of gratitude. Ask yourself whether it fosters more or less loyalty and commitment. It's normal and understandable to find the process difficult - please don't judge yourself. It's brown belt work on the way to Black Belt Husband; it's meant to be challenging.

- In every aspect of life, we can see the goodness in things, or we can see what is wrong. Where is the majority of your focus in life, and in relationships?
- We are evolutionarily wired to assess threats easily. This is how our species has survived through time. But sometimes, the part of our brain that assesses threats is hyper-reactive when it doesn't need to be. To fight against this part of ourselves, we have to be mindful enough to realize that we are not in danger, even though we may feel otherwise. When we're hyper-reactive to threats in relationships, we can be critical or find ourselves looking for an exit. Have you been accused of being critical or looking for an exit?
- Criticism is a derivative of some discontent, just like loyalty is a derivative of gratitude. Have you been accused of being too critical of others in your life?
- We compliment others to the extent we genuinely appreciate them. Is it easier or harder for you to give compliments generously?

- The more appreciative we are, the more we bring loyalty and commitment to our relationships. Without gratitude, exiting is always an option. This usually shows up in threats about divorce during arguments. Is this something that happens in your relationship?
- We know statistically that the grass is not greener as shown by divorce rates for second and third marriages. However, it can be tempting to be allured by the wish of someone better out there. Is this something with which you struggle?
- Maturity in relationships develops to the point where we can experience joy in the thorn bushes that have rose petals. In your life and relationships, do you see rose petals or do you see thorns? If you see thorns, don't judge yourself; just know you can change your thought process by developing more gratitude.

DEVELOPING A MORE BALANCED PERSPECTIVE

Developing more gratitude isn't complicated, it just requires that we give it a little thought and effort. The best way to develop more gratitude in our lives is to take some time to intentionally reflect on and remember what we're grateful for in our lives. The truth is, every one of us reading this book has so much to be grateful for, despite our circumstances. And at the same time, I realize that many reading this book may be going through a challenging time. Being grateful doesn't dismiss life's burdens or challenges. We need to learn to live in the both/and frame of mind as opposed to the either/or frame of mind. Life and all its experiences are never completely good or completely bad. When we're able to see life and all our experiences with a more balanced perspective, we can be sure we are taking strides on our journey to Black Belt Husband. We can honor the difficulties in life and relationships, while simultaneously appreciating the gifts they bring. In blue belt work, we focused on declaring what was important to us with more honesty and assertiveness. In this chapter, we're bringing balance by reflecting on what we already have and our gratitude for it.

BLACK BELT HUSBAND TRAINING: TEN REASONS WHY YOUR WIFE IS AMAZING

I want you to write a list of the top ten reasons why your wife is amazing. Perhaps you're at a place in your marriage where this is a challenging exercise. That's okay, but the exercise is still necessary to arrive at your goal of Black Belt Husband. Your wife has ten really great qualities and characteristics and I can say that confidently without knowing her. It's your job, as an aspiring Black Belt Husband, to be conscious of those things and continually reflect on them. I want you to write down ten reasons why your wife is amazing and commit to reading it every day for thirty days. It shouldn't take you more than a minute and my promise to you is that at the end of thirty days, you'll see her in a whole new light. Grounded in gratitude, it will be a total game changer for your relationship.

GRATITUDE HELPS SUSTAIN US ON THE PATH

Black belts in Brazilian Jiu-jitsu have completed somewhere around ten to twelve years of dedicated and rigorous training. BJJ differs from other martial arts in that black belts are very rare because of the time, effort, and physical demands required for the achievement. Most wash out along the way. The immense challenge and demand of BJJ is what separates it from the pack from other martial arts. There is an incredible amount of appreciation that comes with earning a black belt because the commitment required is so intense.

Undoubtedly, relationships too can be very challenging and require a deep commitment to proficiency and dedication. White belt husbands want to feel all the good of relationships without the necessary change or hard work required. The title of Black

Belt Husband isn't earned easily and the journey to becoming a Black Belt Husband will challenge you, stretch you, and ultimately change you for the better. In the end, you will be very proud of your commitment to the journey. What's more, you will be the beneficiary of all your hard work and relish in the joy it will bring to your life.

At times during the journey toward Black Belt Husband, it may be hard to see the benefits of sticking it out and continuing on the journey. BJJ black belts talk about how many times they thought about quitting. Similarly, you may think about quitting on your way to Black Belt Husband. The thought is natural and predictable. However, when you become more rooted and connected to a sense of gratitude, it will make the challenging moments more tolerable and allow you to tough it out. If you have a hard time with gratitude, your loyalty and commitment will always be in jeopardy. Becoming a Black Belt Husband requires that you reflect on and appreciate the good. Gratitude is the thing that will sustain you along the way.

BROWN BELT SKILLS TEST

PRACTICAL SKILL NEEDED TO MOVE FORWARD

When we're not grateful for what we have, our discontent will always be driving us toward exits in a relationship. An exit is anything that turns us away from our partner. Exits can look like using alcohol, porn, or even leveraging the threat of divorce as ways to disconnect. Exits are the places we go, the things we say, or the things we do when we're struggling with our relationship. Exits can be practical or psychological, meaning we might act them out or simply having a running narrative in our minds. Either way, exits in relationships undermine the necessary security for marriage.

Required Skill: Blocking Your Exits

You know your exits. It's where you escape to when you're frustrated, overwhelmed, and want to run away. It's what you do or where you go when you're pissed. Black Belt Husbands have to be mindful of their own personal exit strategies and fight against them. Spend some time thinking about your own personal exits and write down your top three. Share them with one of your band of brothers to hold yourself accountable for changing this part of your life. To become a Black Belt Husband, you need to challenge your exits, see how they diminish the loyalty and commitment to your relationship. Our goal is to shift from our exits to a mindset of gratitude.

CHAPTER 12

Brown Belt III:
Purposeful; Getting Rooted in Our Why

ALIGNING WITH OUR PURPOSE CEMENTS OUR CONVICTIONS

Black Belt Husbands are purposeful about their personal approach to being husbands. For Black Belt Husbands, being a great husband is much deeper and richer than any temporary positive feelings that may come from a good marriage. Although feeling good in your marriage is important, it's not the primary motivation for Black Belt Husbands. Instead, Black Belt Husbands are driven by a deeper purpose that reflects their calling to live meaningfully and leave behind a powerful legacy for others. Their role as husband is part of the bigger legacy.

Why do we get married? Why is being a good husband important? Beyond the tangible benefits of marriage, the deeper answers to these questions is our declaration for what we really stand for and believe in. What do you stand for? What do you want to be known for when you die? The brown belt journey requires us to think about our bigger purpose in marriage because we can't be great leaders without knowing the deeper calling that's driving us. If we are to be leaders of dimension, we have to be grounded in our why. It is our North Star, keeping us oriented toward what we know to be right in life and in marriage. Our why is our answer to the question, "Why is being a good husband even important after all?" The more we are rooted in the answer to this question, the more we are fulfilled in the marriage journey.

Most people enter marriage because they fell in love and it seemed like the appropriate next step to take in their lives. Inevitably, there reaches a point in all relationships when the decision to get married comes into question. We will experience doubts and fears that leave us questioning whether or not to remain committed to the marriage. The relationship will go through periods when it doesn't feel good and it doesn't serve us well. We might come to places and feel like we've grown apart, or that we aren't in love. In these moments, without a deeply rooted and purposeful why, we are adrift at sea without an anchor. Understanding our why is what sustains the relationship during challenging times.

Marriage can be difficult and if you're reading this book, you know all about it. You will undoubtedly want to quit. Anybody who tells you they haven't had doubts or haven't wanted to quit along the way is not being honest with you. Even the most solid marriages pass through these moments. But one key difference between Black Belt Husbands and other husbands is that Black Belt Husbands are driven by a deeper purpose and understand their why.

Many husbands resign themselves to ending the marriage when things get hard, when they fall out of love, or for a myriad of other different reasons. Black Belt Husbands are not easily shaken by these transient feelings. Black Belt Husbands understand their bigger purpose and their own personal "why". A major aspect of becoming a great leader in marriage is being cemented in your greater purpose.

WITHOUT A "WHY", A SATISFYING LONG-TERM MARRIAGE IS NOT POSSIBLE

Our why is a light that can guide us whenever we feel lost. Without being truly grounded in our deeper purpose about marriage and own personal core values that guide us, we will be swayed by the challenges of life and eventually blown off course. Our purpose provides the grounding we need to be calm and steady, even in the midst of a swirling hurricane. As we become more grounded, we are much safer and more trustworthy as husbands. We're showing the people around us that we are steady, and reliable. That we can be counted on even when things are rocky. There is nothing small about this kind of predictability; it's deeply reassuring to our loved ones.

Over the past twenty years, the marriage counseling community has placed a great emphasis on helping people feel better as a way to keep them from breaking up. Don't get me wrong, I love the idea of more contentment, more satisfaction, and more peace in relationships. Still, the problem is that no therapist can help couples feel this way all the time. What, then, do we do and where do we turn when all the techniques and skills we've learned aren't working?

Even in the best marriages, there are difficult moments that will tempt us to run or check out. There will be times when positive feelings begin to wane. When that happens in spite of learned skills, people can simply chalk up the relationship to a "bad match". The general lack of a deeply rooted why is a core issue in so many troubled marriages today. I'm not afraid to tell people today, "If you're getting married simply to be happy, don't do it".

Getting centered in our why is so important that having a long-term committed relationship without it is impossible. With it, we become similar to that sturdy tree planted deeply in the soil. When the winds come, it does not get toppled over. As leaders in business or marriage, we need to be grounded in a belief system that guides our choices. This is our why.

WITHOUT A "WHY", WE'RE GOING TO FEEL LOST IN THE WILDERNESS

When we lack clarity around our deeper purpose, we inevitably run into problems. Our why is what we represent, what we defend, and what we want our legacy to reflect. When we're disconnected from it, we allow ourselves to be mistreated, do things we regret, and in the end, run the risk of living a life we don't feel proud of. People who harbor regrets during their final days often talk about being disconnected from their why and not living in their deeper purpose. When life presents us with choices and decisions, we look to our why like we would look to the map for guidance if we were lost in the wilderness. Without our why we're left wandering in directions that can be perilous for us.

As brown belt leaders, and soon to be Black Belt Husbands, we simply can't be wandering in the proverbial forest and hoping for success in the marriage journey. Who would follow that kind of leader? I know I wouldn't and I'm pretty sure you wouldn't either. When people are deeply rooted and clear about what matters to them, it helps others around them feel safe. When you have a clearly defined why for your life and marriage, you naturally carry a certain confidence and inspire that confidence in others. When you're not living in your why, your partner simply isn't going to follow you.

Over the course of my career, I have seen three common problems when working with men in marriage: porn, affairs, and alcohol abuse. When I work with guys struggling with these problems, we first tackle the emotional component. What all therapists know is that things like alcohol abuse, affairs, and porn are symptomatic of deeper emotional problems. As the emotional component gets sorted out, we highlight the way the behaviors are out of alignment with their value system.

How these issues are not congruent with the men they want to be.

When we are caught in unhealthy behaviors, we are always disconnected from our core values, and our big why. When we get more grounded and have greater clarity about our own internal values, alcoholism, affairs, and porn stand in stark contrast to the way we aspire to live our lives and the legacy we want to leave behind. We want to be remembered for being great, and these three things are never what we want to be remembered for.

WHAT DO YOU STAND FOR? AND WHAT WILL YOU FIGHT FOR?

Every man has an inborn desire to be remembered for something great. All of us want to be remembered for living full and complete lives. We all want to look back on our lives and feel a sense of satisfaction. It's an existential quality that separates us from other primates. Part of my motivation for writing this book was to give back to my two sons. I wanted to write something that I could offer them as a guide for their own marriage journeys. Even if they never read it, I'll feel just as good knowing I went through the effort to give them something I found valuable. Being a great leader means leaving a great legacy and there's no better legacy to leave than that of being a great husband and father. But to leave a great legacy, we have to begin by living out our core values. We have to get clear about our deeper purpose.

There have been several research articles in the media recently about regrets people express at the end of their lives. It's interesting research because it reveals what is to come for us if we live out our why or if we don't. When asking thousands of men and women about their life regrets, a common theme was wishing they spent less time working and more time with the people they cared about. That's powerful research, because it reflects something we may encounter at the end of our own lives. I'm assuming you're reading this book because being a good husband is important to you and it does align with your deeper purpose. If you died tomorrow, would you be remembered as a great husband who gave his all to his family?

BEING GROUNDED IN YOUR "WHY" SEPARATES YOU FROM THE PACK

If I asked you about your deeper why behind being a Black Belt Husband, would you be able to clearly define it for me? A lot of guys would struggle with this question because they haven't really considered it. If you're like most guys, you got married because you were in love and it seemed like the natural next step. But feelings of love will wane over time. What then? Black Belt Husbands are clear about their why and live their lives accordingly. Our why shapes our decisions and forms a blueprint for our lives. Take some time with the questions below and see what comes up for you. You're at a critical stage of the Black Belt Husband journey.

- Most people in western culture get married because they fell in love, which is great. But that loving feeling will come and go throughout the marriage journey. So how do you justify working on being a good husband when you don't feel in love?
- What does being a great husband mean to you? Why would you work hard on it and what significance does it have beyond the good feelings it brings?
- When it comes to creating the story of your life, did you remind yourself that you are the author and that you write your own character? Sure, you can't control all of the circumstances of your life, but you can control

how you react and respond to them. How do you feel about authoring your journey as a husband?

- What do you want your obituary to say about you as a husband?
- Where do you find your motivation to push and challenge yourself when everything inside you says quit?
- Do you have marriage role models who are really clear about their why?
- How important is it that your children and your grandchildren remember you as a great husband? Are you living your life in a way that moves in the direction of that legacy?
- Every man leaves behind a story about his life. How do you want the story of your life to be written? If the story ended today, how would you feel about it?

DEVELOPING A BLACK BELT HUSBAND MISSION STATEMENT

Getting more clarity on your why for becoming a Black Belt Husband is one of the final steps of the journey. We're nearing the end of our work together and we now need to work on cementing our convictions for being masterful husbands. In our current culture, having convictions and guiding ethics for being masterful husbands can be perceived as an outdated or antiquated form of orthodoxy. Being a Black Belt Husband may come at a cost because you'll likely feel separated from other husbands who may see your steadfastness as rigid. You might be criticized or judged for being committed. Black Belt Husbands believe so deeply in what they stand for that criticism from a postmodern, relativistic culture doesn't sway them.

An effective way of thinking about your why and living rooted in it, is to reflect on your core values and develop a mission statement to which you can turn for guidance, reassurance, and remembrance. Much like a successful business, Black Belt Husbands need mission statements that reflect what they're all about. But before you can craft your mission statement, you have to get clear about your core values:

BLACK BELT HUSBAND TRAINING: MAKING A DECLARATION OF WHO YOU ARE

Our core values are the words that best represent what matters most to us. These core values will drive our mission statement. Think through and list six personal core values ranked in priority order. These six words best represent who you are and how you're uniquely you. Keep in mind that you're creating a working document that gets continually refined over time as we grow.

For reference, here are my six core values in priority order:

1. Authenticity
2. Freedom
3. Commitment
4. Simplicity
5. Meaningfulness
6. Health

Black Belt Husband Mission Statement

Once we've spent some time thinking through our core values, we can spend some time crafting our Black Belt Husband mission statement. A Black Belt Husband mission statement provides clarity about the purpose motivating you as a husband. It defines who you are and how you will live. To help craft your Black Belt Husband mission statement, you can use these five questions (as well as the questions in the prior section) to guide your thoughts:

1. What qualities and characteristics inspire you to become a Black Belt Husband?
2. What do you not want to be associated with about being an average husband?
3. Why is being a Black Belt Husband important to you, as opposed to an everyday husband?
4. What values do you embody that promote being a Black Belt Husband, versus the everyday average husband?
5. Who are other Black Belt Husbands that you respect? And why do you respect them?

Your Black Belt Husband mission statement is an expression of your priorities in relation to your life as a husband. When you write your Black Belt Husband mission statement, you are describing the person you are aspiring to become.

When your Black Belt Husband mission statement is done right, it should be something that you feel passionately about. It has to resonate at a deep level because it's going to challenge you. If you really don't believe it, you'll fall off course. I hope you feel very proud of yourself at this point because you are crafting your legacy. When you have your mission statement finished, print it and post it somewhere you'll see it regularly. Be sure to share it with your band of brothers.

OUR "WHY" BRINGS PASSION AND ENTHUSIASM FOR LIFE

Without being clear on our deeper purpose, we'll never live enthusiastically for anything. The truth is, life is sometimes hard, and relationships are sometimes hard. We can be very proficient at learning skills to improve the quality of relationships, but they will still test us. I've been helping couples improve their relationships for many years; my wife is also a marriage therapist doing the same type of work and even though we have a lot of "knowledge" about how to make relationships work, we still get stuck at times. None of us are immune. Understanding our personal core values will bring laser-like focus to what we do; it is a distillation of the meaning and purpose that transcends difficult moments. The why drives us to live passionately. The reason many men are not passionately living out their role as husbands is because they are disconnected from, or simply don't know, their why. Black Belt Husbands see their role as something much greater than something that revolves around their happiness. Ironically, as we are more connected to our why, we begin to create relationships that do bring us more happiness.

When we are clear about our why, we can move easily into passionate and directed action. Not being swayed by temporal feelings. Confusion around our values always breeds apathy and non-action. Living an apathetic life is misery, and with all the husbands I've worked with in my practice, I see apathy as one of the reasons why so many men are discontent in their lives. When we're apathetic and not living out our purpose, it breeds depression, alcoholism, anxiety, and always leads to some form of a midlife crisis. If we're not living aligned with our core values, then we can't live passionately. And if we're not living passionately, we're not living well. As we get more closely in tune with our personal core values and feel more rooted in our Black Belt Husband mission statement, we discover a greater sense of purpose that extends past our moment by moment feeling state. This deeper purpose drives us to show up in our relationships enthusiastically with the aim to build something great.

When we're passionate about the big picture, we aren't so easily caught up in the insignificant stuff. And when we're not getting caught up in the insignificant stuff, the relationship feels much more peaceful. This new paradigm sets the stage for greater levels of overall satisfaction in our relationships. This is the beauty and critical necessity of getting connected to our why.

BROWN BELT SKILLS TEST

PRACTICAL SKILL NEEDED TO MOVE FORWARD

Most of us never think about our own mortality until we're faced with a catastrophic event that awakens us to the fragility of our lives. When something like this happens, it usually causes us to evaluate everything. In these moments of contemplation and evaluation, we often realize that we're not living our lives with the kind of intention and purposeful conviction that we want for ourselves. These moments of heightened awareness often inspire great life change in people. However, we don't need a catastrophic event to inspire us to reevaluate our lives. We can do it now even while things are going smoothly and even incorporate this type of life contemplation routinely in our lives.

Required Skill: Write your own Obituary

It might seem like a morbid assignment, but it's an important one. If you died today, what people say about you could differ from what you would want them say about you. So, if you were to die today and you were able to write an obituary about the life you want to be remembered for, what would it say? Writing our obituaries reminds us that we are all leaving legacies and that we have an opportunity to leave a great one or an unfulfilling one. Spend a little time writing your own desired obituary in no more than 500 words. Here are some questions to help you think through what you might want it to say:

- What mark are you making on the world?
- What do you want to be remembered for?
- What do you want your family to say about you?
- What do you want your friends to say about you?
- Whose lives are impacted most positively by you?
- What do you really stand for? And what did you really fight for?

BROWN BELT ATTRIBUTES SUMMARY

The brown belt journey is about developing the right mindset and the necessary skills to be the kind of leader that our loved ones happily follow. Too often, men prematurely insist on a leadership position without developing the necessary foundation and framework that is required of any great leader. The foundational skills required for great leadership have been developed in our journey from the white belt through the brown belt. When we develop these attributes through continual effort, leadership flows naturally. Becoming a leader worth following is the final stop on the way to Black Belt Husband. In this last section, we're perfecting three essential qualities: generosity, gratitude, and purpose.

Brown Belt I—Generosity Summary:

Becoming a generous leader is all about moving from a me-centered frame of mind to an other-centered frame of mind. Being other-centered does not mean that we deny ourselves or fall back into the trap of being passive and submissive because we fear conflict. By the time we make it to the brown belt, we know how to advocate for ourselves confidently so that we can freely give from a place of strength. Great leaders are always concerned for the wellbeing of their followers.

Brown Belt II—Gratitude Summary:

Gratitude is a necessary component for the Black Belt Husband journey. Without it, we will be infinitely discontent, spending our time aloof and wondering whether the grass is greener on the other side. When we live from a place of discontent, our loyalty begins to wane. We only look at what's wrong, which erodes the trust and safety of those closest to us. Everything in life can be viewed from a standpoint of thankfulness or discontent. Our vision of our lives is a choice. Black Belt Husbands live from a place of gratitude, which cements their loyalty in marriage.

Brown Belt III—Purposeful Summary:

Great leaders are empowered by a vision and a purpose that exceeds their own self-interest and transient feelings. So too is the brown belt leader worth following. Without a deeper purpose and an alignment with our why, we will only see relationships as self-serving vehicles. As our feelings of happiness wax and wane, as they do in all relationships, we risk letting our feelings direct our lives in a way that is incongruent with our personal core values. Staying grounded in our why is our North Star, guiding us in challenging times.

Congratulations!
You've graduated from Brown Belt!

CONCLUSION

Leaving a Legacy That Matters; Welcome to Black Belt Husband

A brave man, a real fighter, is not measured by how many times he falls, but how many times he gets back up.

—Master Rickson Gracie

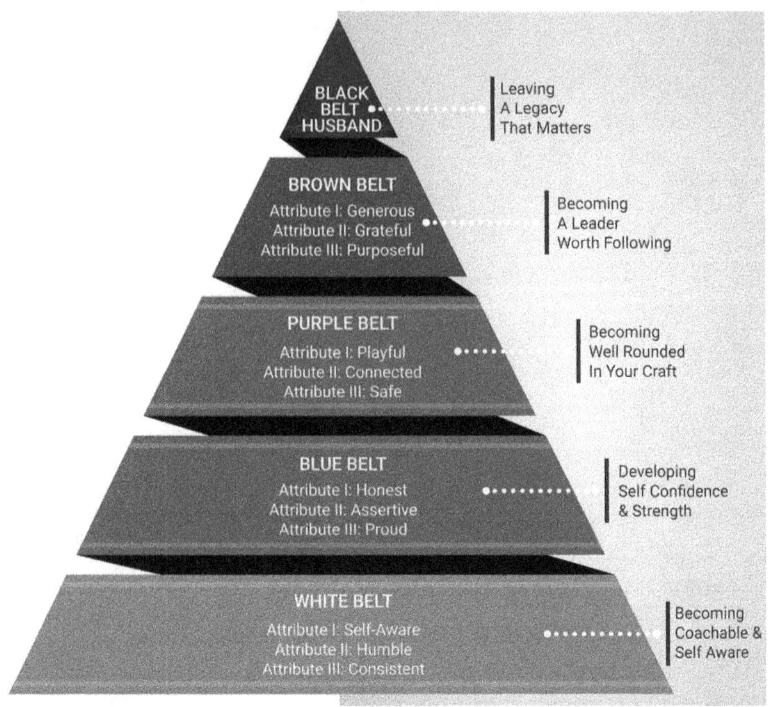

A BLACK BELT IS JUST A WHITE BELT WHO DIDN'T QUIT

Becoming a Black Belt Husband is an incredible honor, and an accomplishment worthy of immense pride. Black Belt Husbands separate themselves from the pack of one-dimensional men by pursuing a positively life-changing, yet challenging endeavor that carries great meaning and fulfillment.

But as much as this book is written about marriage, it's not really a marriage self-help book. This book is about becoming the man you were born to be. It's about becoming the mature masculine man that may be hidden deep inside you, wanting to be discovered. This book is about all of us becoming the men that some of us wished had guided us along the way in our own lives. Becoming a Black Belt Husband is a personal journey of self-discovery and authentic masculine expression. It just so happens that when we embark on this journey, our marriages have a way of transforming themselves.

Wherever you're at on the Black Belt Husband journey, I want to urge you to persevere. I'm not talking about your marriage; I'm talking about refusing to quit on yourself. You are worth every ounce of effort that it takes in this pursuit, and I promise you that the rewards you will receive in the end are worth it all.

I know you are a good man. I know it because you've made it all the way to the end of this book and you've cared enough to stick it out and learn about this Black Belt Husband thing. You already have what it takes and don't think for a second that you don't. They say in BJJ that a black belt is just a white belt who didn't quit. It's no different for the Black Belt Husband process. You owe it to yourself to keep going, no matter how tough it gets and no matter how much you want to quit. You can't quit on yourself.

When I first started training BJJ, it was very humbling and even humiliating at times. I was a BJJ white belt and I used to get crushed. Still, I saw what the black belts were able to do. I was so inspired by their skills that I continued to stick it out through injuries, defeats, and experiences of a bruised ego. On my BJJ journey, there have been discouraging moments when I felt like I was going backwards. My friends and training partners would encourage me, push me along, and tell me to keep showing up. Every now and then I would get a few wins, feel really proud of myself, and realize that I was actually improving.

The Black Belt Husband journey works similarly in that there are times when we will feel like we're not making any progress. This book serves as a guide to keep us on the path for when we feel lost. If we use this material as a roadmap, we will eventually arrive at the rank of Black Belt Husband with a skill set that sets us apart from the rest. That is my promise to you.

THE WORLD IS CRAVING HEALTHY MASCULINITY

The journey toward Black Belt Husband is about becoming a well-rounded, multi-dimensional man. It's about being humble and proud at the same time. It's about being assertive and other-centered together. It's about being honest, and playful in unison. For all of us to develop into the men we were truly meant to be, we need to cultivate the ability to move back and forth between these complimentary characteristics. Our ability to do so affords us the opportunity to employ a wide variety of skills at the right time. Being multi-dimensional is the way of the Black Belt Husband.

In Brazilian Jiu-jitsu, we see how being multidimensional plays out well with black belts. When I train with a black belt, sometimes he will submit me with his assertiveness and remind me that he is the alpha. At other times, he will play with me and allow me to be the alpha. Sometimes he will correct me when I err, and other times he will be affirming and supportive when I'm feeling frustrated. This ability to be multidimensional at the appropriate times is also the spirit of being a great husband in marriage.

More than ever my friend, the world is desperate for men like you to live the Black Belt Husband journey. So many men are lost, confused, and uncertain about what it means to be a good husband and a good man in the 21st century. Masculinity is under attack from people who don't understand what healthy masculinity is supposed to look like. Our responsibility as men is to show the world what it truly means. Black Belt Husband is a roadmap to live out your full masculine potential in life and in relationships.

Wherever you're at on the journey, I want to invite you to be part of the elite group of men who are changing the world in the arena where it counts the most: their families. Although becoming a Black Belt Husband is a proven path to being infinitely more content in your personal life, the Black Belt Husband journey isn't simply about your own personal happiness. The Black Belt Husband journey is about our children and the creation of a legacy that truly changes the world into the future. It's about being a beacon of light in a world that craves to be reunited with healthy masculine men.

YOU DON'T HAVE TO FEEL LOST ANYMORE - THERE IS A CLEAR PATH

The Black Belt Husband journey is a carefully designed and proven system to help us realize the best version of ourselves. From white belt to black belt, every step of the journey builds upon those that came before. Men can use it as a detailed roadmap of where they've come from and where they need to go.

Becoming a Black Belt Husband is so much more than learning simple communication skills or any other commonly suggested tool that is traditionally taught in marriage counseling. The reason these tools rarely work is because the foundation hasn't been laid in advance of using the tool. Or conversely, the tool is too simple for the individual who is much further along in the process.

For example, telling a husband that he needs to be more sacrificial (brown belt work) in his marriage, despite the fact that he lacks the internal strength to be appropriately assertive (blue belt work), would be moving him in the wrong direction. He should not be thinking about sacrificing more until he has developed the self-confidence to assert himself first. Otherwise, the sacrifice will feel forced and will breed resentment. The Black Belt Husband process helps men move from the beginning to the end of the path in a structured and comprehensive way that builds the necessary foundation for success in life and marriage. The Black Belt Husband journey is getting to the roots and working upward from there.

In BJJ, the belt ranking system has tremendous value. From the perspective of an outside observer, it might seem trivial that the practitioners wear different colored belts. I used to think so too until I experienced the gap between myself as a white belt and a blue belt. In reality, the belts are incredibly accurate representations of the skills of those wearing them. The belts are meaningful in BJJ because they show everyone where you are in your training and where you'll likely need help.

Just as the belt system in BJJ serves a very practical purpose, so too does the belt system for Black Belt Husband. It helps us know where we are in the journey. The Black Belt Husband process helps us gain total clarity on our development as husbands and healthy masculine men. If we follow the belt system and commit to being resilient along the way, we will eventually obtain the title of Black Belt Husband.

EVERY GREAT SUCCESS IS THE RESULT OF A THOUSAND FAILURES

I wish I could promise you that the Black Belt Husband process is easy. But if it was that easy, becoming a Black Belt Husband wouldn't be anything special. The Black Belt Husband journey is difficult. I have too much integrity to lie and tell you that it's going to be easy. As you must know by now, nothing worth achieving ever comes easy. With that said, if I can do it after living in a family that didn't know how to do marriage, I know you can do it too.

There is something deep within our bones that relishes a sense of accomplishment in the face of challenge. Men love to be the victors of battles and win by overcoming personal hardships. It seems like it's hardwired into our DNA. I imagine the Nordic Vikings sailing across the Atlantic to the new world. Starvation, dehydration, war, bad weather, etc. were all really good reasons to turn back and give up. But they didn't. They persevered, pushed through, and eventually found a new land worth celebrating. The timeless stories of personal challenge, perseverance, and victory are deeply rooted in our masculine identity and call all of us to its fulfillment.

Even though we seem to be hardwired for great accomplishments through hardships, there is still fear inside us all. That fear will be the biggest hindrance for our achievements. I imagine the Nordic Vikings set sail for a new world a thousand times before they actually made it. There were undoubtedly many hardships and fears that caused them to turn back before they eventually reached their destination. But they persevered and pushed through, knowing intuitively there was something great waiting for them.

The same can be said for our journey to the rank of Black Belt Husband. It's challenging and fear will cause us to want to turn back and give up. But we have tools and a new blueprint that can help us stay on the path. We have our band of brothers to which we can turn in moments of difficulty and accomplishment. We don't have to feel unsure or alone when deciding what to do next. There is a clear map and as long as we tap into our deeply masculine commitment to persevere, we will be the beneficiaries of our own achievements.

BLACK BELT HUSBAND AWAITS YOU

The Black Belt Husband journey offers us the roadmap and necessary skills to develop into the men we are meant to be. And in the process of becoming the men we're meant to be, our relationships get totally transformed. We can have deeper meaning, more intimacy, lasting connection — and hold on to our inner badass as well. We can create a legacy that truly matters to us. However, only a few will achieve this prized title and role.

Will you join me in being one of them?

Visit www.BlackBeltHusband.com to learn more.

www.ingramcontent.com/pod-product-compliance
Lightning Source LLC
Chambersburg PA
CBHW050238270326
41914CB00034BA/1967/J

* 9 7 8 1 7 3 2 4 4 8 4 1 4 *